Women and Health
Cultural and Social Perspectives

Women and Health Series: *Cultural and Social Perspectives*
RIMA D. APPLE and JANET GOLDEN, Editors

The series examines the social and cultural construction of
health practices and policies, focusing on women as subjects and objects
of medical theory, health services, and policy formulation.

Mothers and Motherhood
Readings in American History
Edited by Rima D. Apple and Janet Golden

Modern Mothers in the Heartland
Gender, Health, and Progress in Illinois, 1900–1930
Lynne Curry

Making Midwives Legal
Childbirth, Medicine, and the Law, second edition
Raymond G. DeVries

The Selling of Contraception
The Dalkon Shield Case, Sexuality, and Women's Autonomy
Nicole J. Grant

Crack Mothers
Pregnancy, Drugs, and the Media
Drew Humphries

And Sin No More
Social Policy and Unwed Mothers in Cleveland, 1855–1990
Marian J. Morton

Women and Prenatal Testing
Facing the Challenges of Genetic Technology
Edited by Karen H. Rothenberg and Elizabeth J. Thomson

Women's Health
Complexities and Differences
Edited by Sheryl Burt Ruzek, Virginia L. Olesen, and Adele E. Clarke

Listen to Me Good
The Life Story of an Alabama Midwife
Margaret Charles Smith and Linda Janet Holmes

Travels with the Wolf

A Story of Chronic Illness

Melissa Anne Goldstein

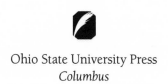

Ohio State University Press
Columbus

Library of Congress Cataloging-in-Publication Data

Goldstein, Melissa Anne.
    Travels with the wolf : a story of chronic illness / Melissa Anne Goldstein.
        p. cm. — (Women and health)
    Includes bibliographical references.
    ISBN 0-8142-0840-1 (alk. paper) — ISBN 0-8142-5043-2 (paper : alk. paper)
    1. Goldstein, Melissa Anne—Health.   2. Systemic lupus erythematosus—
Patients—Pennsylvania—Philadelphia—Bibliography.   I. Title.   II. Women &
health (Columbus, Ohio)
RC924.5.L85 G65   2000
362.1'9677—dc21
[B]   99-089483

Text and jacket design by Gary Gore.
Type set in ITC Berkeley by G & S Typesetters, Inc.
Printed by McNaughton & Gunn.

9 8 7 6 5 4 3 2 1

To my loving family,
especially my parents, grandparents, and brother.

If a thing loves, it is infinite.
—William Blake

Contents

Series Editors'
Foreword

Travels with the Wolf is a truly compelling account of a young woman's coming of age while in the grip of a chronic and at times life-threatening illness. Melissa Goldstein's descriptions of her illness experience, her medical treatment, and the roles of family, friends, and health care providers are uniformly engrossing. Other books in our series have told of health care systems, health care workers, and health care recipients. This volume—an illness narrative—takes a different approach. It is a memoir, written with a distinctive voice and in a distinctive style that we have taken pains to preserve.

There are many lessons embedded in this autobiography. We see the health insurance system with its many failures. We see the strengths and limitations of individual healers—some of whom are sexist, others of whom are simply unable to cope with individuals whose medical difficulties cannot be easily diagnosed and managed.

Finally, we watch the author struggle in her relationships with family and friends at a time in her life when her identity as an adult and as a chronic illness sufferer are emerging simultaneously. All of us live with a sword hanging over our heads, but Goldstein has felt that cold steel blade and written eloquently of its presence and meaning in prose and poetry.

Acknowledgments

When I think of all the people who have helped me and the many ways they gave of their time, expertise, support, and creativity to the project *Travels with the Wolf,* I become overwhelmed at the thought of acknowledging everyone properly. I would need another entire book to do it. So I will just say a deeply felt thank you to all and take a moment to express my gratitude to a few organizations and individuals.

First, I would like to thank the Lupus Foundation of America, especially the Delaware Valley and Philadelphia chapters, and the Arthritis Foundation. Both foundations generously provided source material for the book.

The National Coalition for Independent Scholars was extremely helpful in assisting me after I finished the manuscript. I am indebted to Karen Reeds and Joanne Lafler for their encouragement and savvy professional advice as I navigated the publishing world.

In 1997 the *Pharos,* a journal of the medical humanities, published my essay "Medicine and Poetry: A Pathway of Communication," which was based on a section of *Travels with the Wolf.* The publication of that piece gave me a much-needed test run for my work.

There are several people to whom I must give special thanks. Without them, this book could not have been written. I begin with Charles Rosenberg, for he first encouraged me to combine my personal experiences of and research into chronic illness and turn them into a book.

A writer needs critical readers, and I have been lucky to have an assortment of dedicated readers. Some were colleagues from my field; others were laypeople who read the manuscript out of friendship. I am especially grateful to David DeLaura, Debbie Gaines, Heather Widmayer, and Janet Pisansky.

Though I am a writer, words evade me when I try to express all that Renée Fox has done for me. I have greatly benefited from her vast practical and scholarly wisdom throughout the process of transforming this manuscript into a book. Ever since I conceived of writing *Travels with the Wolf,* she has never wavered in her belief in this book and in me. Her support has been a gift beyond measure.

Joanne Weber and Lee Kovacs also deserve my deepest gratitude. I have lost count how many times Joanne read and reread the entire manuscript. When I was in an especially manic phase of the work, I would call her at any time of day or evening and, with barely a hello, read her revised pages. Not only did she tolerate my calls, but she also gave me essential feedback and critique. Her patience and ability still amaze me.

Lee, a gifted writer, is my partner in this writing enterprise. It so happened that she and I were at work on our books at the same time. We read each other's manuscripts, researched publishers together, and generally kept each other sane throughout the writing and publication process. I know that writing this book would have been more difficult and less enjoyable without her company.

I also wish to thank Robert Klitzman and Liz Rozin, two established writers who took the time to guide a beginner through the writing and publication of her first book. A special word of appreciation must go to Janet Theophano for her loyal friendship. It was she who led me to the Ohio State University Press, where I at last found a caring home for my book.

It has been my privilege to work with the editors at Ohio State University Press. They are professionals who bring enthusiasm, dedication, and kindness to their craft. I particularly want to thank my series editors, Janet Golden and Rima Apple, for all their support. In Janet, my book found a guardian angel.

I must certainly acknowledge my parents, Sandy and Larry Goldstein, as well as my brother, Jonathan Goldstein. My brother and father gave me, among many other things, technical support. My mother was my first reader, the toughest and the most devoted critic I will ever have. All chapters were entrusted into her merciless hands before anyone else saw them.

Finally, let me acknowledge the large community of the chronically ill, their families and close friends, as well as those health professionals who care for them. Before I became ill, I barely knew of your existence. Over these past eleven years, you have graced and blessed me with your stories of your own experiences. I have listened and remembered. Your voices echoed in my head as I wrote every page of this book. So I tried to bear witness for us all, bringing our voices together so that those who know nothing of chronic illness will hear. And understand.

To all the people who helped bring this book into being,

Thank you.

Introduction

Reader, before you begin traveling with me, I should give you some guidance and explanation. In the following pages, I tell a story of myself, my family, my friends, and our experiences with the disease systemic lupus erythematosus, known more informally as "lupus" or "SLE." Lupus, which is a member of the rheumatic family, is a chronic illness of the autoimmune system. It can affect any system in the body, and its effects range from mild to deadly. Though lupus is generally not well known to the public, it is by no means rare. In 1998 the Lupus Foundation of America (LFA) estimated that somewhere between half a million and a million and a half people in the United States have been diagnosed with lupus. That number grows by sixteen thousand each year. We have no idea how many people endure the disease's ravages without knowing its name. The LFA states, "More people have lupus than cerebral palsy, multiple sclerosis, sickle-cell anemia, or cystic fibrosis."

I tell my story through a synthesis of materials and styles. Originally this manuscript was an expansion of my master's thesis about lupus and chronic illness. My thesis advisor had urged me to develop the thesis into a book. But I decided that I did not want to talk about lupus or living with a chronic illness through the medium of a scholarly, academic work. I wanted to find a form that would be more creative, a genre in which I could speak with a voice that was both literary and scholarly, a way of communication that would reach a broader audience.

I found my form and voice by intertwining the themes and insights from my thesis with my poetry. Throughout the book, I use my poetry to illustrate my meaning and explore my deepest emotions, moving in and out of poetry and prose to produce an integrated whole. Some of the poems were written during the period with which they are associated in the book, others later. As one of my literary heroes, William Wordsworth, explains, "I have said that Poetry is the spontaneous overflow of powerful feelings: it takes its origin from emotion recollected in tranquillity." I usually needed time to reflect on my experiences before putting them in poetic form. The white heat of emotion produced the initial notes and images, but the final poem could not be written until I was tranquil and objective enough to apply intellect, skill, and craft to the raw feelings.

Besides my poetry, I have included materials from various sources. Being the ultimate pack rat, over the years I have saved copies of letters I wrote to my family, friends, and physicians. I also kept letters sent to me. I have medical summaries written for my many visits to doctors; appointment books; and copies of test results. I kept my diaries as well. I interviewed family members and friends to gain their perspectives and refresh my own memory. I have attempted to incorporate all these kinds of information into the book. As best I could, I have tried to produce a work that was true to my own, my family's, and my friends' experience.

For reasons of privacy, I have changed the names of family members (except for my parents and brother), of friends, and of all the health-care professionals who have treated me. My names for my characters are in keeping with the ethnicity, age, and personality of the individual the name is meant to represent. A few of the names are symbolic; I will leave you to decipher their meaning. I also omitted or changed the names of the hospitals where I was treated. The identity of the institution is not important, only what took place there.

As I worked on my manuscript, I discovered that in the writing, the book took on a life of its own. No matter how many outlines I produced ahead of time, when I finally put pen to paper (or fingers to keyboard), I found that I often headed in a different direction from the one I had planned. One new thought led to another. In the morning I rose eagerly, curious to see where my writing would take me that day. So the writing became a journey in itself. When I finally reached the end of the book, I realized that I had come a long way from my thesis. I had created a work that contained more than the story of my illness. For this book is a tale about myself and my family, a story about becoming—my becoming a young woman, a writer, and a teacher.

Now it is time for us to be on our way. Take my hand, and let us travel on together.

Prologue

Summer 1995

TELL ME about your lupus from the time you first became ill to the present," said Dr. Kearney, a specialist I was consulting for a second opinion. It was August of 1995, the summer when *Travels with the Wolf* was conceived. How often I had given physicians my medical history. Over the past seven years, I had grown accustomed to the expectations of health-care professionals. I knew what information to provide and how to convey it. After listening attentively, Dr. Kearney examined me, then ordered lab work. At the end of the visit he promised to call in a few days with test results and suggestions for possible treatments.

My mother and I left Dr. Kearney's office. I think she had been looking forward to the appointment with equal anticipation. I had excellent medical care in Philadelphia, but even aggressive treatment had not controlled my illness, systemic lupus erythematosus, a chronic disease of the immune system. We both hoped that Dr. Kearney, with his fresh perspective, might be able to offer helpful advice.

As the train sped away from Manhattan, my mother and I grew quiet. She soon fell asleep. Rocked rhythmically by the motion of the train, I began to drift, neither sleeping nor waking, and found myself alone in a borderland where my thoughts were my mode of travel. I began my journey by thinking of the story I had just recounted to Dr. Kearney and the illness narrative I would soon begin to write. For some time I had wanted to write such a narrative, yet I had always felt, and continued to feel, an inexplicable resistance to beginning this project. Why?

I carried this question with me as I roamed the borderland, finding no

1

answer, no way to lay the question aside. Finally I stopped my wanderings in frustration. Much to my surprise, I saw that a mountain had risen up before me, splendid with grassy slopes and peaks draped in a pure white mantle of snow. I knew this mountain. It was the mountain of good health. I had been trying to ascend it for seven years. I had thought that only when I had gained its heights could I look down and behind to chronicle and understand my illness experiences. But I had failed to climb the mountain and so thought myself a failure. Why would I want to expose my shame to others? I was waiting for the moment when I could write as someone who had triumphed over her disease.

That is what those who had come before me had done, or at least so it seemed from the multitude of books given to me by family members and friends who meant well. In these memoirs the courageous heroes and heroines use their moral and spiritual strength to cure themselves of their disease. Where did that leave me? How could I give voice to my own narrative within this narrow framework which ultimately defines the value and worth of a life, of a person, in terms of achieving and maintaining good health?

I stared at the mountain, dreaming of the pleasures I might find at its summit and in the valley of good health that stretched outward from its base. That valley was hidden from me as I stood in the desert of chronic illness on the other side of the mountain. But then I spotted something I had not seen before. A road wound its way through the desert. The road, heading east, rose and fell, preventing me from gaining a clear view of its path. Straining to see, I recoiled from the harsh desert sands. But, there in the distance, I saw intimations of blue shimmering waters, mysterious and inviting, deep and peaceful, relieving the sting of the desert sun. I also glimpsed what looked to be a river, flowing east, parallel to the road, both road and river disappearing at the horizon's edge. I set my feet upon the road and did not gaze back at the mountain. I found that I had left my question behind me and put an answer in its place. I would not wait for remission to write my narrative. I could not. It distorts the experience of living with chronic illness to do so, for chronic illness does not disappear, even with the abating of symptoms. It becomes a part of life and self in both subtle and more obvious ways. My tale is complete in its incompleteness; that is the essence of chronic illness.

As I left the borderland and arrived in Philadelphia, I found that I had gone a great distance. Now I could begin.

PART I

1
Shifting Sands

December 1996–February 1997

Y OU'RE NOT in school. You're not working. What do you do with
yourself all day. Stay in bed?" With these words, Dr. Hornbach, a doctor I barely knew, addressed me, his tone accusing as he entered the
room and planted himself in front of me. I lay on the hard gurney shocked
into muteness. I stared up at Dr. Hornbach. He had a broad build with the
solidity of granite, an immovable object cloaked in white. From his height
of over six feet, he looked down at me, his craggy face and ice-chip blue
eyes showing no compassion. His eyes clearly did not see me the way I and
others thought of me—as a twenty-seven-year-old writer, a poet, and a
young woman who despite the ravages of disease had retained her identity,
dignity, and femininity.

Chocolate brown framed in thick, dark lashes, my eyes are my most
noticeable feature. I am fair-skinned with a rosy bloom on my cheeks, a
peaches and cream complexion as a friend of the family always comments. I have long, abundant, wavy auburn hair with red highlights. At
five feet two, I continue to mourn my lack of height, as well as the weight
gain and the round face bestowed upon me by steroid treatment. But I
take consolation from having what people describe as a radiant smile,
ebullient laughter, and a mellifluous voice. In Dr. Hornbach's cold, probing stare, however, I saw nothing more than a defective specimen that
had the temerity to present itself for his inspection. He watched me,
unmoved and unmoving, judging me while the sheets entangled me as I
shook helplessly with the violent tremors that had in part brought me to
the ER.

My parents and I had arrived in CGH's (Community General Hospital's) ER at 10:30 that morning, February 1. When I was taken back to the treatment room, both my parents accompanied me and remained by my side. The nurse entered the little cubicle and commented, "You look just like your mother. Anybody ever tell you that?" Many people have remarked on the resemblance. My mother has recently become a red head, though her hair used to be brown, similar to mine. Her hazel eyes are lighter than my own, but their shape is the same. I see my smile, my nose, the contours of my face in her. When she speaks, I hear my own voice; people often mistake us for each other over the telephone. We match in height, and like me, she has always tended toward plumpness. In our cheerfulness and optimistic natures, we are also kindred souls.

Some have said I look like my father. We share certain mannerisms and expressions, but there, I think any physical resemblance ends. My father's complexion is olive, and his hair is jet black. Behind his glasses, my father's eyes are dark brown, but in their lighter shade and almond shape they differ from mine. I also did not inherit his dimpled smile. Though he did give me his genes for being short. He stands at about five foot six, and he is on the portly side.

Later that morning my aunt Beth, my mother's sister, came to the ER and stayed with us the entire long day. She had been notified through the family network that my parents and I were in the emergency room. There was never any question that she would come, as she had in many other times of crisis. In the cubicle where my family and I waited for hours, there was a telephone. Constantly it rang as love and concern from extended family traveled over the wires and filled the small room.

I had been in a lupus flare for the past several months, beginning in December. On Christmas Eve I had spent nine excruciating hours in the ER of the large teaching hospital where I had received my care for the past seven years. I can still remember, with the clarity of a vivid nightmare, those black, uncushioned metal chairs in the waiting room. The chair's unyielding surface pressed into my lower back, which already sizzled with pain. I had lost some sensation in my hands and in the lower part of my body, from my waist to my toes. Earlier in the week, plates had left glaring red marks and even blisters on my fingers as I had obliviously pulled hot dishes out of the microwave. Beneath the numbness in my legs, though, I felt as if a legion of tiny rats gnawed relentlessly, producing an aching, continual pain. Wearily, I arose every ten minutes to visit the ladies' room, attempting, but almost unable, to urinate. I was feverish and trembling. Nausea washed over me in bile-green tides.

Occasionally I broke out into myoclonic attacks in which my hands, arms, legs, and even my head would jerk or spasm uncontrollably, sometimes violently. My face, including my eyelids, also fluttered and tremored. Sometimes only my face might be involved, just one side of my body, or single limbs. As I shook, a little girl, maybe about four or five years old, pointed at me and said loudly, "Mommy, why is she doing that?"

I knew that she was only a child. I should not be angry or hurt by her understandable curiosity. But at that moment she seemed cruel. I felt humiliated enough by my spasms. I wanted to snap at the little girl, "I'm not doing this on purpose. If I could stop it, I would. I'm sick. Why don't you mind your own business anyway!" I did not feel comforted when the mother, blushing scarlet, told her daughter to be quiet. The mother then moved herself and her daughter to another part of the room, careful to avoid meeting my eyes as she passed me.

After several hours of waiting, teary from pain and exhaustion, I told the triage nurse, "I can't sit up any longer. I'm ready to lie down on the floor." An hour later she placed me on a gurney, which was no softer than tile. At 5:30 in the morning, after I was finally examined and had blood drawn, I was discharged by an intern. "You've got a bladder infection or a lupus flare. Not sure. Don't know enough about lupus. You need a rheumatologist. We can't find one. You don't want to be here over a holiday anyway. Go home and follow up with your regular doctor. Here's an antibiotic just in case you do have a bladder infection."

After that visit to the ER, my mother stayed with me in my apartment for a few days. Always optimistic, I hoped that my symptoms were due to a bladder infection, which antibiotics would cure. I thought that I was feeling better; the rest, the antibiotic, and the pampering from Mom seemed to be helping—or so I convinced myself. The following weekend I had holiday plans I intended to keep. My friend Rachel, whom I had known since we were both in the third grade, had bought us orchestra seats to a Broadway show, and I had organized dinner for eight in a New York restaurant.

The group consisted mainly of college friends who had settled in the New York–northern New Jersey area. We all kept in close touch by telephone and e-mail, and I was greatly looking forward to seeing them again. I had missed the brunch one of my college friends had given the weekend before because of what I thought was a stomach flu. I had promised my friend I would not miss this dinner. There was also someone in whom I was interested, and this was my chance to find out if our friendship could become something more. I was determined to have this day and evening in New York and not permit the disease to steal it from me.

The train trip to New York was uneventful. But I was still having bladder problems, a situation that worsened as the day progressed. Our theater seats were up a flight of stairs in the middle of a row, and the ladies' room was on the other side of the building, two flights down. I missed most of the show as I traveled back and forth, returning to the ladies' room every fifteen minutes. The ushers and bathroom attendants shook their heads in sympathy each time I reappeared. As the day wore on, I wore out, the rats tearing at my legs, the fire blazing in my back.

After the show we took a taxi to the restaurant. We passed several hospitals along the way, and I wondered if I should stop at a local ER. In the past, I had relied on adrenaline and willpower to push the disease aside as I finished my work or socialized with friends and family. I thought I could call up enough of that strength to pull me through this evening.

We were the first of our group to arrive at the restaurant. As I looked over the elegant dining room; the exquisitely fashioned, artistic desserts set on the tray; and the fresh salmon, lobster, and shrimp glistening on their bed of ice, I burst into tears. I left a shocked Rachel standing by the hostess, then rushed to the ladies' room. In eighteen years of friendship, I do not think she had ever seen me cry.

I went into the stall and pulled the door shut behind me. My tears of fury, disappointment, and frustration soaked the tissues. I knew I could not last through the dinner. My drive and desire to continue on were not enough. Not tonight. I was spoiling the evening for myself and my friends, especially for Rachel. Guilt and shame pierced through me like an icy blade. A few minutes passed, and I rejoined Rachel. Pasting a smile on my face, I said, "Can we catch the first train home?" She did not question me, but consulted the train schedule and called a cab from the restaurant.

Once we reached Penn Station, we dashed over to the conductor. We explained the situation and begged him to allow us to get on the sold-out, overbooked train that was leaving in a few minutes. The next train to Philadelphia was not for another hour and forty-five minutes, and I could not have sat in the station that long. I had just enough strength—maybe—to board the train at that moment and drag myself home. Otherwise I would have to go to a local emergency room. The conductor studied us a moment. We must have appeared frantic, because without a word he kindly escorted us onto the train and into the dining car, the only place with two available seats.

The rest of the trip home was spent mostly in tense silence. From time to time Rachel would ask how I was feeling, and I would reply that I was all right. I smiled as I spoke, trying to reassure us both, but my smile felt false and plastered to my face. I knew I was not fooling either of us, but if I had moaned and groaned or catalogued my ills, it would not have made the pain and discomfort disappear. I felt that I would only become more of a burden to her, and I had given her trouble enough for one day.

Later, Rachel commented that my silence had frustrated her, making her feel uninformed and helpless. "What if you had passed out, and I had to take you to an ER? I wouldn't have even known what to tell them was wrong, except that you went to the bathroom a lot." So many times in the past, my efforts to shield the people in my life backfired, only causing them hurt or more anxiety. I had tried to change—and had improved. But old habits born out of personality and experience are difficult to completely break.

Once again Mom came to my center-city apartment, but this time she took me home with her to Doylestown, a suburb of Philadelphia. I was too sick to remain alone in my apartment. From December to January the lupus burned through me, and in January we flooded my body with high doses of oral and IV steroids as well as chemotherapy in our attempts to damp the fires.

The only brief respite came when a friend from my undergraduate years visited me in Doylestown. Sang attended medical school in Chicago. He was currently on winter break and, for the month of January, was staying with his family in New York. Though we often spoke on the phone, we had not seen each other for the past few years. In July he would begin his internship, and it would only become more difficult after that for us to meet. But twice I had to cancel because of infusions or medical tests. Finally we had only one chance to get together before Sang went back to Chicago, and although I still felt ill, I wanted so much to see him that I told him he was welcome to come. I was still moving in the slow lane, I said, and could not offer too much in the way of excitement. He assured me that he did not mind.

We spent a wonderful few days together. From the moment he walked in the door, he never made me feel guilty or embarrassed for not being able to entertain him the way I would have liked. When I needed to sleep during the day, he contentedly read a book, played with the cats and dog, or talked with my mom and dad. He did not need to be waited on; if he was hungry or thirsty, he went to the kitchen and fixed himself a snack or took a drink. When I was awake and alert, we enjoyed long conversations, played Scrabble, and watched many videos. Sang was restful and easy to be with. For him my company was pleasure enough. With gentleness and grace, Sang accepted my illness and offered me the gift of true friendship.

On a Sunday at the end of January, a week after the chemotherapy, I returned to my apartment, though not without trepidation on my and my parents' part. My father felt that I was making a mistake. My mother was anxious as well, but she knew how eager I was to return to my normal routine, and she wished that for me, too. She wanted me to continue with my work and be with my friends. So she set her worries aside, reassured my father, and went shopping. Being a Jewish mother, she took comfort in stocking my apartment with plenty of food and supplies.

I felt ambivalent. I yearned to go back to my apartment, my little nest on the seventeenth floor and resume the life in which I took such pleasure. Yet I wondered whether or not I could cope on my own. When I pictured my empty apartment, I felt frightened. What if I had yet another crisis? I would be alone. Should I stay with my parents for another week?

Then a voice rose out of the depths of my mind. It was my inner voice that spoke to me with pure honesty. The voice asked, "Melissa, why do you want to stay in Doylestown? Is it because you're really not physically ready to go back? Or are you afraid?" Honesty demanded that I answer "Well, I'm on the borderline of being able to take care of myself. And I'm scared." The voice answered, "The chemotherapy should kick in within a few days after you arrive home. You'll be feeling stronger, not weaker. Remember what your brother told you." And I did. He said, "Melissa, it's natural and normal for you to be frightened sometimes with all the illness puts you through. The only thing that matters is what you do with your fear. You've always gone on with your life. That's true courage."

Anxious, proud, and eager, I packed my bags and returned home. Two days later I attended a meeting at Laurel University, from which I had received a master of liberal arts degree two years before. I hoped that the professor in charge of the meeting might be willing to give me the name of her literary agent. Since graduating from Laurel, I had been working on my book, a narrative of my illness experiences. I had just completed the first draft of the manuscript and was eagerly trying to find a publisher. Though I felt exceedingly ill and unsteady on my feet, I dragged myself to the meeting, feeling a sense of triumph and excitement that I was able to keep the appointment.

The next day, still hoping that I could maintain my regular schedule, I felt a small surge of energy and decided to catch the apartment shuttle downtown, where I would go to the bank and the post office. I had a letter I had written to Professor Esther Stein, my mentor at Laurel, who was spending the year at Oxford. I made my way from my apartment to the lobby, my legs encased in braces, my hand tightly grasping my cane. I was surprised by my weakness. When the bus came, I was barely able to step off the curb and haul myself onto the bus. As the bus moved through the city, I sat in fear. What if I did not have the strength to get off?

Soon my stop came into view. I thought surely I could manage at least the post office, which was in the building just in front of me. Then I would catch a cab and return to my apartment. Cautiously and with difficulty, I stepped off the bus. I walked unsteadily a few feet, then stopped. I realized I was trapped. I had neither the strength nor the balance to continue forward or go back. Would I be able to hail a cab and get myself home? What should I do? I stood, irresolute, petrified. Fortunately, the bus driver had not yet left and had seen my dilemma. He got off the bus, came over to me, and asked if he could assist me into the building. "No, I think I better go home." He helped me back on the bus, then off the bus when we reached my apartment. A neighbor saw how shaky I was, grabbed my arm, and walked me up to my place. I never left my apartment again that week until my parents took me to the ER.

The day after I attempted to go to the post office, I was no better, only weaker and more tremulous. So I called Dr. Averapporti, my rheumatologist and the specialist in charge of my care. Such a call was no simple matter. It involved six steps. First I spoke with the secretary. She gave my message to the nurse, who telephoned me back and talked with me. The nurse then relayed my message to the doctor. He gave her instructions for me. Finally, the nurse called me again and told me that Dr. Averapporti felt my weakness might be related to my steroids and that I should decrease my dose slightly. I felt as if I had just played a game of "Telephone" or "Whisper Down the Lane." Did my doctor understand the extent of my weakness, or did my message become minimized as it got passed along? My internal alarm bells were not easily triggered, but they were all pealing.

I spent the next few days mainly going from my bed to my bathroom. When I felt adventurous I would go into the kitchen to try to feed myself. Walking with two canes, I lurched around the apartment. If I fell, I did not think I could get myself off the ground. I kept my portable phone by my side in case of emergency. It was difficult to get out of a chair, dress, bathe, or even feed myself. As I tremored and shook, food went flying off utensils, and buttons slid out of my shaky grasp. The shower was a serious danger zone in my current state. When I felt my best I could manage to shower, but I needed to rest for several hours before and after. By the end of the week, I could no longer function on my own.

On Saturday morning I could bear it no longer, so I telephoned the rheumatology service. The resident told me to go to the ER. I replied, "That's fine. But when I went in December, no one from rheumatology was available. The entire visit was a waste of time. I *will not* go through that again. If I go to the ER, I expect someone from rheumatology to meet me there." He agreed. I called my parents, who took me to the hospital in a wheelchair. Otherwise we would have had to call an ambulance.

At the ER, after my parents and I were ushered into the treatment room, hours passed. Doctors and nurses flowed in and out of the room, but they were all strangers. My regular rheumatologist, Dr. Averapporti, and my regular neurologist, Dr. Fields, were not available that weekend. First came the general house staff, who conducted their own examinations. They summoned the neurology resident to assess my tremors and weakness. She tapped reflexes, tested sensation, and watched me shake and stumble as I walked. A frown creased her face as she said, "These tremors and weakness don't match a neurologic pattern, and your weakness doesn't seem to be caused by your steroids. You have to be on a higher dosage of steroids for a longer period of time. Let me read your chart, and I'll talk to you later."

Several hours later, Dr. Hornbach and his shadow, a resident who spoke not a word, appeared. After his first obnoxious questions, he continued, "Well, your blood work shows no evidence of infection or lupus flare. I think we'll send you home soon." My parents were flabbergasted. My mother answered, "How can we bring her home? She can't live on her own in her apartment. She can't come to our house, because she can't climb the steps. And the bathrooms and bedrooms are on the second floor."

The rock looked at my mother as if she were auditioning for a part in a remake of *Mommy Dearest*. "You mean you don't *want* her at home?" Trying to control her temper, my mother replied, "It's not a question of not wanting her at home. She's not physically able to function at her place or mine." Dr. Hornbach responded, as if making a great concession, "Well, we could admit her." But then he added accusingly, "She's not really that sick. What if insurance won't pay for her to be in the hospital. What'll you do then?" My mother answered, "We're triply insured, and the hospital will get paid." As he walked out the door, Dr. Hornbach rumbled, "Well, we'll see. I'll speak with the other doctors, and we'll come back."

My family and I could not believe what was happening, though previous encounters should have rendered us immune to surprise at this kind of treatment from a doctor. The minutes ticked slowly away, melting into hours heated by our anger and frustration. By late afternoon my parents were considering taking me out of CGH by ambulance and going either to another hospital or back to their home in Doylestown. The ambulance drivers could carry me up the stairs of my parents' house.

As I lay listening to my parents plan to take me away, I felt panic, almost terror. How could I leave what had been my safe port? I had received my care at CGH for so long, and over the years had forged close relationships with several doctors, especially my regular rheumatologist and neurologist. I had always thought of the people at CGH as family. I had been hospitalized many times here and was often in the building for outpatient appointments or treatments. I knew many of the attending doctors, interns, residents, nurses, physical and occupational therapists, secretaries, lab technicians, housekeeping staff, and transport personnel (who wheel patients around the hospital)—all the people who come together to form the hospital community. I was friendly with the hospital newspaper seller, a round little man with two missing front teeth and a charming, quirky smile. We always exchanged comments about his business, the weather, and my health.

Despite severe, crippling disease, much of the time, I was able to go about my daily round. I attended college and graduate school, and eventually embarked on a full-time writing career. All the while I enjoyed an active social life; I dated and delighted in spending time with friends and family. My ability to journey forward came out of an inner security, part of which was a result of feeling that should the disease go beyond my ability to handle on my own, my hospital family would welcome me and enfold me in their protective arms. They could not offer me a cure, but they could and did give caring, capable, and reliable treatment. I was not alone with my disease. But if I left my hospital family, I would wander, lost in the desert of my illness, unaccompanied by the doctors I had known and trusted.

I loved my own family, and they provided all the support they possibly could, but they had no professional medical knowledge or resources. Their love was not enough to fight the illness, as they had learned years before. I told my parents to wait, to give the doctors at CGH a chance. "You know what they're going to say. That it's all in your head, and you're just being hysterical," Mom snapped, her fury directed not at me but at the medical system that was withholding treatment from her suffering child for whom she could find no relief.

Mom's worry about the doctors' dismissing me as a hysteric came from hard experience. And the last time it happened was still fresh in her mind.

In October, a few months before this latest flare, I had been hospitalized at CGH for evaluation of the seizures for which I had been treated during the past few years. Throughout the week I spent in the hospital, the epileptologist, Dr. Gresley, witnessed many myoclonic spasms, but nothing my family or I would have called a seizure. The episodes I considered seizures had been seen by nurses, family, and physical therapists, but never by a doctor.

In my follow-up appointment, Dr. Gresley stated that the myoclonus looked "atypical" and that she was troubled by my cheerful disposition. Perhaps I was burying deep-seated concerns about my illness and converting them into physical symptoms. A few months of psychotherapy should uncover those hidden feelings and end the myoclonic attacks. As for the seizures, since she had not witnessed one, she could not comment about their type or cause. I left her office enraged. How many times would I have to hear the same excuse? Because the physician could not pinpoint the source of my symptoms, I, through my supposed diseased psyche, must be to blame.

As for therapy, I had been seeing a psychiatrist for several years. Dr. Averapporti, my rheumatologist, was also—initially—concerned about my cheerfulness. Though, knowing the burden chronic illness places upon the patient, Dr. Averapporti mainly wanted a psychiatrist to provide me with some emotional support. The psychiatrist, Dr. Cohen, and I had spent a couple months getting to know each other. Dr. Cohen admired my upbeat personality and considered it an asset, not a sign of abnormality or emotional illness. After a few months he had discharged me, saying, "Consider me a friend who will be here to listen when you need me." Taking him at his word, I would visit him several times a year, usually after a lupus flare. After all, the mind and the soul need to be ministered to as well as the body, for the disease affects a person, not a collection of organs. In Dr. Cohen's office I found healing of a different kind from that gained through the wonders of pharmacology or the skill of a surgeon's knife.

Though I did not see him regularly, Dr. Cohen was my psychiatrist. I became even more infuriated when I thought of Dr. Gresley's supreme arrogance in making a psychiatric diagnosis without even consulting the psychiatrist who had known me for the past several years! I decided to go to Dr. Cohen for advice. I told him Dr. Gresley's conclusion, not hiding the fact that I was extremely upset and insulted. But I trusted his judgment; if he felt there was any possibility that she was correct, I was perfectly willing to begin regular psychotherapy with him. It would be a

small price to pay for ridding myself of the myoclonic attacks and seizures—which were debilitating, sometimes painful, and humiliating.

But Dr. Cohen shook his head. "I looked for signs of psychosomatic
illness when you first came to see me. As you know, your cheerful nature
worried your doctors and made them think you might be denying the extent of your disease. But, as I've always told you, your sunny disposition
and optimism is your strength and a part of you. It's certainly not patho-
logical. I saw no evidence of psychosomatic illness several years ago, and
I see nothing now which indicates an emotional cause for your physical
symptoms. You have serious physical, medical problems." He paused a moment, to add weight and emphasis to his next words. "If you have a doctor
who is dismissing your physical disease, then you need to find yourself
another doctor."

After consulting with Dr. Cohen, I felt greatly reassured. I then discussed Dr. Cohen's evaluation with Dr. Fields, my neurologist, and Dr.
Averapporti. My doctors both seemed satisfied with Dr. Cohen's assessment, so I put Dr. Gresley and her nondiagnosis behind me, considering
the whole experience an unpleasant but finished piece of business. I had
no idea that her pronouncements about my seizures would affect me so
profoundly months later, poisoning my relationship with other physicians
and generally compromising my medical care.

Like my mother, I, too, wondered and worried about whether or not I
would be labeled as a hysteric once again instead of being treated. The day
seemed to be heading in that direction. Still, I hoped that I would receive
appropriate care. When I thought of the alternative, I felt trapped, cor-
nered. I was physically helpless. I needed medical treatment from somewhere, and I needed it immediately. If I went elsewhere, I would have to
wait for the first available appointment, usually a delay of a month or two.
I imagined going to another institution and beginning again. Maybe I would
find competent care, maybe I would not. CGH had not been my first stop
for medical treatment since I had become ill almost nine years before. I
knew what was out there. And even if I found skilled practitioners, I would
be dealing with strangers who did not know my complicated history; they
would be at a terrible disadvantage. I put my faith in Dr. Averapporti and
Dr. Fields. Surely they would come and take control of the situation. So my
family and I continued to wait.

By this time it was 5:30, time for my next doses of medicine. My
mother informed the intern. An hour later, I had not yet received the medicines, which were supposed to be taken on a strict schedule. My mother

again asked the intern about the meds. Irritated, he barked, "The medicines aren't up from pharmacy yet. Melissa will have to wait and so will you. You know, there are a lot sicker patients in the ER than Melissa. And I won't stand here and listen to you criticize me, neurology, or rheumatology." (Up to that point we had said nothing negative about the intern. We also had not complained about my medical care or lack of it to him or any other doctor that day; he must have overheard us talking.) My mother completely lost her composure. Her face flushing to a color almost matching the red of her hair, she yelled, "I never criticized you. And if this were *your* daughter, *your* sister, *your* mother, or *your* grandmother, would you be telling her and the rest of your family to 'just hang in there?' I don't think so!" With that, she stomped off to my apartment to bring me my medicines.

Aside from releasing some of my mother's pent-up tension, I thought that screaming at the intern was basically useless. After all, he had no real power. But word must have gotten out that the patient and family in cubicle seven were not satisfied customers, because ten or fifteen minutes later, the emergency room chief, Dr. Marshall, paid me a visit.

Dr. Marshall was an older man in his fifties with a kind, gentle, and unhurried manner. He introduced himself to me and my family, shook our hands, and gave my father his card. He turned to me and said sincerely, "I'm sorry you're not feeling well. Would you mind if your family stepped out for awhile, so we could speak together alone?" My family filed out, and Dr. Marshall came to sit beside me on the gurney. He spoke in quiet, sympathetic tones, "I understand your parents are worried about you. If you were my daughter, I'd be concerned, too." His gaze was warm; his demeanor was authoritative without being bullying or overbearing. The effect was calming; I could easily imagine this man as someone's father. An image flashed into my mind of him carrying an old-fashioned black bag as he made his house calls. Did I somehow associate gentleness and concern with an era in medicine's past? Perhaps his soothing presence just seemed out of place compared to the general callousness, indifference, and rudeness that had surrounded me all day.

Dr. Marshall continued, "Obviously something brought you into the ER on a Saturday. You had an appointment with your neurologist on Monday, but you felt too sick to wait. Tell me why you came to us. How is this different from your usual symptoms? People who have lived with chronic illness for a long time usually know their bodies better than the doctors. Chronically ill people also often have some idea of what can be done to alleviate the problem. What's wrong, and how can we best help you?"

He meant what he said; his attitude was not patronizing or condescending. I spoke for awhile, and he listened intently, occasionally inter-
jecting questions. We even discussed my manuscript. He was genuinely
enthusiastic. He repeated the title of my book several times so that he would
recognize it when he saw it in the stores.

By this time, it was about 7:30 in the evening. Dr. Marshall ended our
conversation by forming a plan of action. "Do you trust your regular rheumatologist and neurologist, Dr. Averapporti and Dr. Fields?" he asked me
seriously. "Yes, I do." I assured him. "Well, you've been here long enough.
The doctors have to make up their minds and decide what to do with you.
Right now, you can't be treated as an outpatient. You don't need to visit one
doctor one week and the other doctor the next week. Meanwhile, each
one prescribes different medications while they both write memos back
and forth. You must be admitted. I also want Dr. Averapporti and Dr. Fields
in your hospital room, both of them appearing together, at the same time
Monday morning. They both must put their heads together and figure out
what's happening to you."

Later I learned that Dr. Marshall called both Dr. Averapporti and Dr.
Fields at home, insisted I be admitted, and demanded that both doctors,
together, be in my hospital room on Monday. Dr. Marshall even called both
doctors again on Monday morning to guarantee that they were going to pay
me a visit as they had promised. Once I was discharged from the ER, I was
no longer Dr. Marshall's responsibility, but he cared enough to follow up.

During this flare I met certain individuals I have come to think of as
guardian angels. Dr. Marshall was one of them. Without his intervention I
do not know what would have happened that day. Probably my family and
I would have departed from CGH and never come back. As Dr. Marshall
left the room, his white coat rustling like wings, I lay quietly in the peace-
fulness he left behind. For the moment, at least, I was safe from the gaping
pit, the void which had threatened to swallow me should I have had to leave
CGH. I understood that my problems were far from resolved, but I had
been given hope. Dr. Averapporti and Dr. Fields, two doctors in whom I
placed my complete trust, would arrive on Monday and be able to help me.
All the pieces of my medical puzzle would fall into place, and I would be
treated. My hospital family would not betray me. In a short time, my life
would be my own again.

I could not have been more mistaken.

2
Obstacles in My Path

February 1997

B Y NINE o'clock that Saturday night I was transferred from the ER to a hospital room. When the house staff, an intern and a resident, came in to examine me, I at once saw a familiar face. The resident was a young woman named Amelia (a name I remembered because I thought it so lovely), and she had been an intern when I had been hospitalized a few years before. She knew me immediately, but she did not recall the illness or the symptoms that had brought me into the hospital when we first met. What had stayed in her mind after all this time was my having been a graduate student at Laurel University, my particular areas of study, my writing, and some people we knew in common. To her my illness was not the most memorable or important part of me. I had never wanted my disease to define me, and obviously, with her, the lupus did not. After Amelia left, I smiled to myself. Even in the midst of a debilitating flare, I felt I had won a kind of victory over my illness.

But my sense of peace lasted only through the night. Morning brought back Dr. Hornbach and his almost invisible resident. Dr. Hornbach bluntly informed me that I was in the hospital only because he was so graciously catering to my and my parents' hysteria and inability to cope. If we had not made such an unnecessary fuss, I would be at home. I better not expect any new medications; the lupus had been appropriately treated, and the only thing I would receive was emotional and physical support. He saw in my chart that I was followed by Dr. Cohen, and he wanted Dr. Cohen to talk with me, for it was very likely that these tremors were psychosomatic.

I met this uncompromising statement with my own. "If you want to send Dr. Cohen here to give me emotional support, then that's fine with me. This has been a difficult, painful flare, and tending to my mind as well as my body is responsible medicine. But if you're bringing Dr. Cohen in here because you've decided that I'm a hysteric, then that's completely different. I'm tired of doctors using psychosomatic illness as a convenient label when they don't know what's causing a problem. I won't tolerate it." Hornbach replied, "Everything is psychosomatic," grunted, and clumped out the door.

My visit with the neurology team, all strangers, did not improve my day. The attending neurologist examined me quickly and rapidly fired questions at me, asking how my neurologic involvement and even my lupus diagnosis was reached. She listened to my answers with a skeptical look on her face, then turned to her team and said, "Do we even know she has spinal cord involvement? Does she even have lupus?" As they shuffled out the door, I could not believe what I just heard. Were my basic diagnoses being called into question? Did the doctors now think I was manufacturing every one of my symptoms?

I spent the rest of Sunday and Monday morning waiting for Dr. Averapporti and Dr. Fields, my court of last appeal. The house staff were acting as if I were a psychiatric case. They seemed less interested in my physical symptoms than in my history with Dr. Cohen, continually bringing up his name, and saying that they would try to get in touch with him.

Early Monday morning, the general medicine attending, Dr. Kotler, spoke to me in the hallway. To fight the weakness and stiffness that had only grown worse as the hours passed, I had decided to take a walk with my mother's help. As I walked a few feet down the hall, I put part of my weight on the cane in my right hand, and I leaned heavily on my mother, who tightly grasped my left forearm. I tired quickly. She soon needed the support of the railing to keep us upright. Then I stopped, clinging to the railing on the wall because my legs, arms, neck, and even my head were tremoring so violently I could not continue walking. As I was trying to keep my shaking body from landing on the floor, Dr. Kotler, pointedly ignoring the tremors, asked, "Who are your regular doctors?" "Dr. Fields and Dr. Averapporti," I answered. "Do you see anybody else?" he probed.

I knew what he was after, but a stubborn, angry part of me refused to give him what he wanted. "Oh, I've been to so many doctors here. I've visited at least fifteen departments over the years." I rattled off a few names, but not the one he was pushing me to say. "Don't you see Dr. Cohen?" I explained that I did not visit him regularly, but, yes, he was a member of my health-care team who offered me emotional support when the lupus flared. Dr. Kotler studied me carefully and said, "Well, Dr. Cohen isn't on call. But we ordered a psych consult. Dr. Martin should be coming by later."

I had met Dr. Martin five years before. He was the head of psychiatry at CGH and a friend of Dr. Cohen. Dr. Martin mainly performed psychiatric evaluations, not psychotherapy. It had been Dr. Martin to whom Dr. Averapporti had originally sent me to make sure that my smile and laughter were real and not a mask or a hiding place for grief. I felt immediately comfortable with Dr. Martin. He is a down-to-earth, practical, no-nonsense doctor who also possesses compassion and empathy. In his opinion, I was coping extremely well. He considered my cheerfulness a natural part of my sunny disposition, not a sinister cover or a sign of maladjustment. Nor did he conceive of my optimism as a detriment to my physical and emotional well-being.

Dr. Martin was ready to discharge me when I asked if he could refer me to someone who offered psychotherapy. I liked the idea of having someone to whom I could unburden myself when the illness seemed especially hard to bear. I wanted an objective person who stood outside my circle of family and friends. A person I would not feel compelled to protect by keeping silent or making jokes about the lupus. I wanted a place where I could freely discuss my illness experiences and feelings about the disease when I felt the need. Dr. Martin had referred me to Dr. Cohen.

After a resident informed my mother and me that Dr. Averapporti and Dr. Fields would not be coming early that day, Mom decided to get something to eat and run a few errands. After she left, Dr. Martin arrived. He greeted me by showing me a poem typed on a single sheet. "Do you remember this?" he asked, smiling. It was a poem of mine, "The Weaver." In one of our sessions he had asked if he could read some of my work. I gave him some poems related to my illness, but at the last moment, I included one poem not about illness. I wanted him to see that I could write about more than just lupus.

It was that poem, "The Weaver," that had captivated him. In fact, he requested my permission to use it in a seminar he was teaching. His students were psychiatry residents, and Dr. Martin felt that the poem could help his students learn about the process of denial. I looked at the poem in his hand and was delighted to see that the paper was well-worn and smudged. This poem had not gathered dust in a file drawer over these past five years. Strangers I did not know and would never meet had read my poem, endowing it with continued life and strength. As Dr. Martin held the poem out to me, I recalled the words I had written.

> She is a weaver,
> spinning all day and night,
> creating delicate, glittering deceptions
> which she lays gently about her life
> like new slipcovers
> to place over that which is ugly or faded.
> She drapes her artistry
> over her children and husband.
> Four people who share food, a house,
> but little else
> become a loving, devoted family
> in her eyes.
> She's been spinning so long
> she forgets the shoddy, shabby things that
> lurk underneath her marvelous tapestries.
> If her silken covers slip to reveal the
> bald, bare patch underneath,
> she quickly spins something new
> to lay over the empty spot.
> She is a dedicated weaver.

Like Amelia, Dr. Martin did not view my illness as the central and most identifiable part of me. As he offered me back my poem, I saw myself through his eyes. He showed me the writer.

Dr. Martin and I had a pleasant chat. He wanted to know how I was spending my time now that I had graduated. When I talked about my book and my life as a writer, he was enthusiastic and supportive. He also wanted to know if anything remarkable, other than my flare, had occurred over the past two months. Had I experienced any crises of good or bad fortune? I replied that no, nothing particularly unusual had taken place. He seemed satisfied with my answers. He ended our visit by shaking my hand and wishing me the best of luck. I assume he found no psychiatric pathologies or abnormalities, because he never came back or recommended further psychiatric evaluation or treatment.

And still I waited for the two doctors I really needed. My mother returned. We sat, our tension making the atmosphere thick and heavy like the air in the minutes before a thunderstorm. At 2:30 Dr. Averapporti and Dr. Fields walked in, one right after the other. Dr. Fields came alone, but Dr. Averapporti was followed by a flock of med students and interns. With a smile on my face, I turned to the flock and politely, though firmly, ordered them all out. "I've been speaking with a lot of people these past few days, and the only ones I need to talk to right now are Dr. Averapporti and Dr. Fields. Nothing personal, but I want you all to leave." Dr. Averapporti looked slightly shocked. I had never done anything like that. When at CGH, I always understood that I was in a teaching hospital; I knew what being a patient in such a hospital meant. In various ways, I had played a role in teaching the younger staff members and students. But at this point, my priority was my own welfare, not medical education.

My faith in Dr. Averapporti and Dr. Fields was not misplaced. Within ten minutes they diagnosed steroid toxicity as the cause of my severe tremulousness and weakness. Both doctors noticed that my pupils were fully dilated, and my heart was racing. Dr. Fields explained, "It's as if you're on a continuous adrenaline surge. Your body is on overdrive." We devised a plan to treat the shakes while reducing the steroid dose. Both doctors agreed that I absolutely required in-house rehabilitation. In my case, that meant intensive physical and occupational therapy. Dr. Averapporti wanted me to stay at CGH so that he could personally regulate my medications while I was recovering. Dr. Averapporti would send rehab medicine in to consult, and if they agreed, I would be admitted into the rehab program by Wednesday at the latest. Though the inpatient rehab medicine unit was located in the hospital, it was a separate administrative entity. To move to rehab I would have to be discharged from CGH, then admitted into rehab.

Dr. Averapporti left the room to rejoin his flock, and Dr. Fields followed him. Dr. Fields had been my neurologist for almost five years, and during that time I formed a close relationship with him. He was never an effusive doctor, though his demeanor and manner were always gentle. He had a dry sense of humor and a sharp wit, but I always felt his compassion and empathy. Before Dr. Fields departed that afternoon, I remember him giving me a warm smile and putting his hand on my shoulder in a gesture of caring, concern, and support. Probably that gesture is etched so deeply in my memory because of later events which have rendered the moment bittersweet. For though I had indirect contact with Dr. Fields during the rest of my hospital stay, it was neither gentle nor compassionate. And after that Monday, I never saw him again.

Later that day, a friend of mine, Jean, telephoned. I had met her while we were both in graduate school, and she, too, was writing a book. When I told her what had happened, Jean exclaimed, "I knew you were headed for a crisis when we saw each other on Tuesday at the university."

Jean explained, "I don't know if you noticed, but at the meeting, I was distracted and quiet. You were scaring me! It was your eyes. I never saw anything like it. Your pupils were so dilated there wasn't any brown left. I was watching you when we were sitting in the conference room. Even under those bright fluorescents, your eyes didn't react to the light. Your pupils stayed fully dilated. It was weird.

"I noticed you shaking when you tried to eat that rice bar. When we left the building, you needed me to hold on to you as you got off the curb. We've walked around the city together, and you're intrepid! You've never needed my help. My first thought when I saw you was that you were over-medicated on something. I wondered what on earth the doctors were giving you. I knew you were in trouble. I wanted to say something and go home with you, but I know how independent you are. I was worried you'd be offended." Jean, who is about my mother's age, added, "Besides, you have one Jewish mother. I didn't think you needed another."

I was utterly shocked. And furious—though not at Jean. This woman, who had no medical training, had correctly diagnosed my problem as some kind of drug toxicity five days before I went to the ER. If a layperson, just by being observant and using common sense, could reach an accurate diagnosis, why did the "experts" experience such difficulty? Why were almost three days wasted by the physicians who, after examining me from tip to toe and extracting copious amounts of blood, could come to no better conclusion than that my symptoms were psychosomatic? Dr. Marshall had mentioned the possibility of drug toxicity, but his voice was drowned out in the general cry that I was a hysteric. My anger simmered for awhile, then cooled. For my own sake, I resolved not to dwell on my anger. I had limited strength and energy, and I needed to reserve them for recovery.

Later that Monday afternoon, Dr. Machcinsky and his resident, Dr. Keating, came from rehab medicine to evaluate me. They examined me with skilled hands, offering their concern and kindness through words and touch. They emphatically agreed that I needed in-house rehabilitation and were as eager to work with me as I was to begin my rehab with them. They made a number of suggestions that sounded as if they would benefit me immensely.

Dr. Machcinsky mentioned that I would probably need to stay in rehab for two to three weeks. He also brought up the idea of using a scooter, a kind of motorized cart, at home after I was discharged. I nodded to both the length of stay and the suggestion of a scooter, but I thought to myself, "Now that we know I'm reacting to the steroids, we'll treat the toxicity. Then I'll just need four or five days of rehab, and I'll be back to my usual self, able to settle into my normal routine. I certainly won't need a scooter. I know myself better than they do." I had registered for a literature class at a local college. The class began in a little less than two weeks, and I assumed I would be there. I was looking forward to the intellectual stimulation and to the possibility of meeting eligible, single men.

The next day I realized that there was a complete shift in attitude from the house staff and the attendings. Dr. Cohen's and Dr. Martin's names—as well as any mention of psychiatry—vanished from our conversations. The doctors interacted with me differently. Dr. Kotler became extremely solicitous. But it was more than that. It was as if a gap had closed between me and the doctors. Before, I felt that they were placing me at a distance, weighing and measuring all that I said, because I was not a reliable source. The words I spoke had to be reinterpreted; the physicians assumed that my meaning was distorted because of my supposed emotional illness. But now that my problems were understood to be physical in origin and not caused by a psychiatric disorder, I could be trusted, and my symptoms somehow became real and legitimate in a way that they were not considered before. As I said to my parents when they visited that afternoon, "Well, it looks like I've been taken off the fruitcake list!"

At least I was no longer viewed as a crazy woman. But my battles were far from over. I traveled several thousand miles to Europe and even hundreds of miles across the Arctic with fewer hassles and red tape than I experienced when I attempted to transfer to the rehab unit located five floors below me. There were two issues—bed availability and insurance coverage.

The first obstacle presented itself when Blue Cross and Blue Shield (BCBS), our primary insurance carrier, refused to pay for rehab, a service covered under our contract. At BCBS an anonymous doctor, a paper pusher who had never spoken with me or examined me, pronounced, "Her problems are chronic; therefore, she will derive no benefit from rehab. It would be a waste of time and money. Reject!" Dr. Machcinsky and Dr. Averapporti appealed the decision.

During the appeal process, Dr. Averapporti and Dr. Machcinsky, as well as their staff, bombarded BCBS with phone calls, faxes, and letters. Dr. Averapporti and Dr. Machcinsky spoke with the highest medical personnel in BCBS, to no avail. My parents became involved. Dr. Machcinsky encouraged them and gave them the name and address of the business director of BCBS. My father faxed a letter in which he described the situation and asked for the director's assistance. My father was ignored, too.

At this point, on Wednesday afternoon, it was clear that BCBS was not going to pay, or at least not at a rate rehab was willing to take. BCBS was willing to pay for a few days at a "subacute rate" far less than rehab actually charged. Dr. Machcinsky did not want to set a precedent with the insurance companies by letting them get away with such a tactic. He was a relatively new director of rehab, and he was struggling to build his department. He felt rehab needed and deserved what he was charging, and he would not take less. Meanwhile, without the intensive rehab, I lay in bed and grew weaker. The health of Dr. Machcinsky's department was more important than mine.

I was feeling a growing sense of desperation. CGH wanted to throw me out because insurance had stopped paying for my hospitalization on Monday. Only the stubborn insistence of Dr. Averapporti was keeping me in the hospital, though even he was beginning to talk about sending me home with round-the-clock nursing as well as visiting physical and occupational therapists until this situation could be resolved.

We all knew I needed aggressive physical therapy, which could not be given at home. Dr. Averapporti also wanted to keep a sharp eye on changes in my medication. I thought with horror, "If I go home with the kind of treatment they are suggesting, God only knows when I'll be back on my feet." My mind drifted back to the first time I had extensive rehabilitation. In 1990 I suffered a completely disabling flare. I could not walk, get out of a chair, or even stand without falling. Yet after six months of intensive rehab, I beat my physical therapist in a game of tennis. Seven years later, I could almost feel the racquet in my hand and hear the satisfying "thwock" as I hit the ball, a perfect backhand shot. My legs and arms obeying me once more, answering the orders of my brain, nerves, and muscles to produce strong, fluid motion. Graceful. Healed.

It had been six years since I had played tennis. I knew that aggressive rehab would probably not put me back on the court, but it could return me to independent living. Freed—not trapped, utterly dependent on others. On Wednesday, when Dr. Machcinsky informed us that BCBS was no longer a payment option, my parents mentioned that we were triply insured. My having two other insurance policies was news to Dr. Machcinsky; he was under the impression that BCBS was my only carrier. When he

investigated, he found that the person in the rehab office who was process-
ing my paperwork had overlooked my other insurance, wasting days. The
rehab office would now begin the paperwork for insurance carrier number
two. I put my grandfather on the job of contacting insurance company
number three. My grandfather in Florida, my Zaide (Yiddish for grandfather), had been in charge of all the paperwork for my medical bills. I
wanted to know whether or not insurance company number three would
pay if number two rejected my claim.

My grandfather telephoned back within the hour. "The case worker,
Margaret, a very sympathetic woman, was in tears when she heard about
your problems. She guaranteed that their company would pay, as long as
the other two insurance companies sent her letters stating that they denied
the claim. Here is Margaret's phone number. Let Dr. Machcinsky call her,
so she can tell him herself."

Thursday morning, Dr. Machcinsky did speak with Margaret. But her
verbal assurance of payment was not enough. He wanted it in writing. A
bed in rehab had just become available. Dr. Averapporti walked into my
hospital room as Dr. Machcinsky and I were talking. When he learned the
current status of the insurance, Dr. Averapporti said in exasperated and
frustrated tones, "You know you're going to get paid. You have a free bed.
Put her in it and deal with the insurance later!" Dr. Machcinsky refused.

Friday morning, the secondary insurance company approved my stay
in rehab, and a bed was available. My parents came to see me on their way
to the airport; they had a business meeting in Chicago and would be back
on Sunday. Dr. Machcinsky appeared while they were visiting and assured
them that I would be in rehab later that afternoon. Relief pervaded the
room. Now my recovery could begin. I wished my parents good luck, and
they promised they would call me in rehab that night.

But at 4:30 that afternoon, a resident delivered the news that someone
in the rehab office had mistakenly given away the last few beds. I had the
insurance coverage, but nowhere to go.

When my parents called early that evening and discovered that I was
still in the hospital room where they had left me, they were distressed and
appalled. Mom wanted to fly back immediately. Dr. Machcinsky happened
to come by at that moment. He spoke with both my parents and convinced
Mom to remain in Chicago. He apologized profusely. My father expressed
his anger about how my care was being handled. My father, a mathematician, had received his B.A. and M.A. from Laurel University. Always a loyal
and proud Laurel graduate, my father stated flatly, "After the past week,

for the first time, I'm ashamed to be a Laurel alumnus." Dad informed Dr. Machcinsky that he intended to contact the highest authorities, including the university's board of trustees and its president, and take whatever other actions were necessary to ensure that I received the appropriate care. Dad described himself as "CGH's worst nightmare."

Instead of reacting defensively, Dr. Machcinsky answered sincerely, "A large part of the problem has been BCBS, and I've had more grief from them than all the other insurance companies combined. But I'll also take responsibility for mistakes I made in filing the paperwork and not accepting the subacute rate BCBS originally offered. I hope you'll be as aggressive as you can in advocating for Melissa. I may get into some trouble when you do, but I'm willing to take whatever comes if that will help Melissa. Since I've been head of the rehab department, I've tried to make the hospital aware that there aren't enough beds in rehab and that there are difficulties in trying to get people admitted. No one has listened. Maybe now they will."

After spending almost forty-five minutes on the phone with my parents, Dr. Machcinsky left. Soon after, Dr. Averapporti paid me a visit. He assured me that he would not allow CGH to throw me out over the weekend. He was thoroughly disgusted with the way the rehab business office had mishandled my case. The person who had done my paperwork and was also in charge of bed assignment now had a reprimand in his or her file. General Medicine, of which rheumatology was a part, filed a general complaint against rehab. Looking worn and harried, Dr. Averapporti eventually wished me good night. He left, and silence descended. But it was a fractured, disturbed quiet in which I found no peace, only a troubled anxious sleep.

On Saturday my mother's parents, who lived in Philadelphia, were supposed to visit me, but a violent snowstorm kept them away. I lay alone in the room. My thoughts roamed, wandering into dark places where illness, bureaucrats, and pain reigned, and I was powerless. Outside the snow swirled, oversized flakes coating the streets, the grass, and the buildings. As the day passed, the snow descended so fiercely it obscured everything. The world turned white outside and in, until I was a mere speck consumed by whiteness.

> White-jacketed healers
> walking in white corridors,
> visiting patients wrapped in snowy sheets.

Vast spaces devoid of color
fill this place.
I wear my own clothes,
midnight blue, forest green,
but the vivid hues
seem to fade in Arctic expanses.

Yet it seems to me
that I should find colors
shrieking out
loss, pain, triumph,
shocking pink and deep violet.
Sickness and its experiences
are not all dressed
in muted, sedate, pale attire.

Then, I reconsider.
Perhaps white is the proper color
in this house of ills and care.
For it is the color that is deceiving
in its seeming emptiness.
In its clarity it contains
all other colors of the spectrum,
just as illness comes clothed in
angry purple,
golden yellow.

Looking,
one perceives how
the solid white splinters,
refracts through the prisms
of all the personalities here,
creating a chaotic, brilliant, sharp,
soft human compendium of color.

Though for some eyes,
the vivid array is too harsh and bright;
they will not see.
In their gaze, the hospital remains only
a world of white.

I lay in bed, my eyes closed, almost completely drained. But I gathered my strength to search my inner landscape for the blue sky, the home of the eagle, which I had first envisioned when I was ten. I had been given an assignment to write a poem which I was then asked to read in front of the class. I had written a haiku about an eagle. In my shyness, I trembled before the class. I read the little poem, my eyes glued timidly to the page. When writing the poem, I had imagined, very intensely, with all of my senses, an eagle floating in the bluest sky; I had tried to translate that image, with all its substance, emotion, and color into the poem. When I finished my recitation, there was silence, then loud applause. I looked up to find my fellow students and teacher smiling at me in understanding. They had shared the eagle with me. Through the power of words and poetry, I had connected with them in an entirely new way. I had discovered the wonders and glories of language and artistic expression.

But in the image of the eagle soaring in the blue sky, I had found more than poetry or a way to profoundly communicate and join myself with others, though that was enough to alter the course of my life. Eventually the image became a way to make contact with the Light. Here I pause a moment. I hesitate to speak of this, to lay this bare before you, for fear that I will lose the Light in the telling. And it is such a basic part of me now that losing it would leave me like the ocean bed without the sea or the earth separated from the sky.

Throughout my growing up and into my young adulthood, I felt and hoped that, despite the suffering, evil, ugliness, and chaos that abound, the essence of the world was composed of order, goodness, beauty, and meaning. I could not be certain. I asked many questions and found no definitive answers. But every so often, I thought I caught a hint. . . .

Only several years ago, when I first encountered the Light, did these feelings about the nature of the world coalesce into a firm belief. The Light is the physical embodiment of all that I had sensed, and a great deal more, which I had vaguely intuited. The Light is my faith. I call upon it when the emotional or physical pain of my disease becomes unbearable. And it is through the image of my eagle that I join with the Light to find comfort.

As the snow fell on that day of pure winter I turned inward and upward. I found sky of the clearest blue, the sky of the eagle, the blue of communion. I began with words. I looked to the sky with all that was in me. "Please be with me in my illness. Do not leave me alone in this terrible place." Then the ambient Light descended, washing in waves over me, and through me. I heard whispers, words of solace and healing. They were in a language beyond my conscious translation, but the sense of peace they brought me was total and complete. As the Light poured into me, filling me, I no longer spoke in words. For I was in the Light, part of the Light. I was Light. I did not need words to be heard.

Gradually the Light faded into the most gentle of summer twilights. Soon the sky returned to azure. I opened my eyes knowing that I could call upon the Light again when I was in need. For it is in me; it is outside of me. It is of the world's core. I do not travel alone, for I journey with knowledge of the Light.

Later that Saturday, my brother telephoned. He always seems to know when I need him. Perhaps my brother was sent to me. I tried to crack my usual jokes and make serious conversation about his work and my writing, but after awhile, the tears I had kept inside me during the week escaped. What if I could not get into rehab? How long would it take me to heal? What if the lupus flared again? This time, I suffered almost as much from the treatments as the disease. When would my life assume some semblance of normality?

Jonathan listened and soothed with words of support and practical, common sense. "I know you want to stay at CGH, but if you can't get into CGH's rehab, there are others in the city that can help you. I know you're going to get through this and back on your feet. You've been in worse flares, and you've recovered. You'll do it this time, too. I *know* it. Not because I believe in the doctors or the medicines, but because I have faith in you. I only wish I could be there. I hate being so far away."

I wished he could be in Philadelphia, too. He lived in Wisconsin, at least for the next year and a half, while he finished his Ph.D. in computer science at the University of Wisconsin in Madison. I smiled when I thought of Jonathan, my younger brother by two years. We are such different people in looks and temperament. He has dark brown hair that curls at the ends, especially when it grows longer, and sea-blue eyes which change color depending on what he is wearing. His skin is the reddish-brown of a Native American. My brother is taller, at about five feet ten, than the rest of our immediate family. His build is average, and he is neither overweight nor skinny. My father is a mathematician and a computer scientist, and unlike me, my brother inherited my father's talent and enthusiasm for numbers and computers. My brother is a true free spirit who does not allow himself to be constrained by schedules, rules, and others' expectations. I am more regimented in my approach to life, liking organization and some structure, and I worry more than he does about what others think.

Our close relationship still occasionally surprises me when I think back to our childhood. We did not even like each other much until we were both in high school. My mother used to ask in exasperation, "Don't you two love each other at all?" The only thing my brother and I could agree on was that the answer to that question was "No!" I remember the family going on a car trip to New England when I was about ten and my brother eight. My parents finally placed a suitcase between us to separate us and prevent us from arguing. My mother used to say, more in hope than in certainty, I think, "Someday you two are going to appreciate one another." She turned out to be right.

Finally it was Monday morning. Time to take action. My hospital room was mission control center with Mom manning the phones. Mom had consulted with her cousin, a physician, who was shocked when he heard about the events of the past week. To my astonishment, my mild-mannered, conservative cousin advised Mom, "Just refuse to leave. Don't let Melissa budge out of that hospital bed. They can't toss her out. If they try, call in the press and your lawyer. Here's my beeper number. Call me if you need me." Mom walked into my room at eight o'clock in the morning, and despite her lack of sleep, she was wired awake, and ready for battle.

Dad's post was at home. He called our family lawyer, who contacted the ombudsman, the official mediator, at the hospital. Dad and our lawyer decided not to take any further legal action in the hopes that everything could be settled amicably. Even I became involved. I wrote a letter to the CEO of Community General, who is also the dean of the medical school. I dictated it to Dad, who then faxed it to the dean's office. I felt that everyone was advocating for me, but I wanted to speak up for myself and make a contribution. If nothing else, it would serve as a chance for me to express my indignation at not receiving proper care. My telephone rang constantly as friends and relatives checked the front for the latest news bulletin.

Meanwhile my physicians were appealing to the highest level of hospital administrators and medical personnel. My doctors were meeting at noon, when they would decide what to do with me. Mom was ravenous, having eaten nothing for breakfast before she dashed out of the house at 6:30 that morning. So, at noon, she went to get some lunch, taking advantage of the temporary lull in our attack as the doctors held their conference. Each minute lasted at least an hour as I waited, my most frequent occupation these days, it seemed.

A few minutes after Mom left, a man knocked on the door of my hospital room and introduced himself as the hospital chaplain. Thinking that there had been some mistake and that he was looking for someone else, I replied, "You know, I'm Jewish. Are you sure you're in the right room? My name is Melissa Goldstein." He smiled and answered, "I came to talk with you, if you don't mind." I welcomed him. I explained that I was waiting for my doctors to tell me whether or not I would be admitted to rehab. Though I did not say it aloud, I knew that I definitely was in need of some comfort and distraction.

The chaplain generously provided both for the next hour and a half. His accent was unusual, musical. When I commented on it and asked where he was from, he laughed and explained that he had grown up all over the world—in Africa, Europe, and Canada. He considered himself a citizen of the world. We spoke about traveling, other cultures, and embracing all that people of other nations, traditions, and religions had to offer. We exchanged philosophies of life, and our conversation ranged across many topics, but not the subject of illness.

The burden of waiting was lightened when shared. As at so many other times in my life, when I truly needed help, it arrived. My mother feels sure that this is the result of my dead great-grandmother, Bubbe Ella, her grandmother, looking out for me and protecting me. (Bubbe means "grandmother" in Yiddish.) I had been close to my great-grandmother; I was her first great-grandchild. Even now she sometimes appears in my dreams, looking young and well. She holds my hand and, in her heavily accented Yiddish-English, invites me to talk to her about myself and the family. I always awake from our conversations feeling rested and peaceful.

While the chaplain was still with me, Dr. Averapporti walked in. The chaplain did not leave my side until he heard what Dr. Averapporti had to say. "You'll be admitted to rehab no later than this evening. At least that's what rehab is telling us. Though I'll believe it when I see it." At this point, though I was relieved, I shared Dr. Averapporti's skepticism. I would consider myself admitted to rehab when I was lying in a bed on the rehab floor. Dr. Averapporti and his crew filed out while the chaplain stayed behind. We spoke a few parting words, and he wished me luck. I never saw him again, but I remember him with gratitude. Bubbe Ella, if you sent him, thank you.

Soon after, Mom returned from lunch, and I told her the good news. Mom was cautiously optimistic. Like Dr. Averapporti and me, she would reserve the celebration for my actual arrival in rehab. Throughout the afternoon and into the evening, doctors from rehab and general house staff from the hospital floor poked their heads in to reassure me that I would really be going to rehab that day. Superstitiously, I refused to pack my bags until transport arrived to take me down. But at eight o'clock, my nurse came in to tell me that transport would be coming in ten minutes and to get ready. We had won. If not the war, then one battle.

3

Abandoned in the Desert

February 1997

I begin with this invocation:

> **May my pen be the confessor of sins, and you, my reader, the priest. May the doctors who are in need of it find mercy and absolution in our efforts.**

I DID NOT notice much about my new environment when I finally reached rehab that Monday evening. In my exhaustion, both physical and emotional, faces and objects blurred and ran together like sidewalk chalk pictures on a rainy day. I answered the standard admission questions by rote, changed into my nightgown, and fell sound asleep, more relaxed than I had been for a week.

The next day began at 6:30 A.M., when a nurse entered to take vital signs and wake me and my roommate so that we could get washed, dressed, and prepared for the day, which commenced with breakfast at eight in the dining room. Promptly at eight, a nurse came to wheel me to breakfast. My roommate, a woman in her sixties who was recovering from neck surgery, also left for the dining room, but she pushed her own wheelchair. My wrists and hands were too weak for me to do the same. As I was taken to the dining room, I watched many of the patients, most of whom were over sixty, propel their wheelchairs down the hallway. I felt ashamed that these people, my grandparents' age, were more independent than I.

The dining facility, which also served as a games and recreation room later in the day, was a large, sunny space. A quiet hum of conversation filled

the room as patients conversed with the ease and familiarity of long acquaintance. That first morning I met Jane, a woman in her late forties, who
suffered from diabetes; both her legs were amputated below the knee. As if
presiding over her own table at home, she introduced me to the others. She
asked me when I arrived, what brought me to rehab, and when I thought I
would be leaving. Those were always the first questions posed by an established patient to a newcomer. It was equivalent to a person at a cocktail
party asking another guest what he or she does for a living and how he or
she knows the host. In a few days, I became the established patient and
welcomed newcomers in the way that the unit had taught me to do, performing the many other rites and rituals of the place without even thinking
of or even noticing them until much later.

The rehab unit was organized like a small community, and its residents bonded together much more quickly than they would have on the
"outside." Time took on a different, more intense quality here. We all had
different medical problems. We came from various races, religions, backgrounds, and age groups, but in our common struggle to regain our independence, recapture our lives, and return home, we were the same.

For the rest of the day I was whisked from one session to the next. After
breakfast came physical therapy (PT) for an hour. The physical therapist,
Annie, spent that first day evaluating me, measuring my physical strength,
weakness, and range of motion. Then Annie made a treatment plan based
on what she observed. She decided that I needed to use a walker with
wheels at the front. A rolling walker could be pushed, and I would not have
to pick it up with each step. Though I appreciated the added distance I
could cover with the assistance of the walker instead of the cane I had previously used, I looked on the walker's ugly, bulky frame with distaste. I was
only twenty-seven; this walker belonged to an older person, not to me.

From PT I was taken to occupational therapy (OT), where my hand
strength, coordination, sensation, and ability to perform basic tasks of
independent living were assessed. The occupational therapist, Samantha,
though always called Sam, wheeled me back to my room, where I collapsed,
worn out. But my rest lasted only a few minutes. Time for lunch, served
promptly at noon.

The afternoon flew by as I went from one therapist to another. I returned to PT for another hour. Later I was brought to recreational therapy.
Though my expression remained polite, I thought to myself, "This is
degrading. I have a master's degree. What are they going to have me do,
weave baskets?" I was soon sorry for my haughty attitude. The recreational

therapist, Judy, was a delightful young woman who described her role as assisting patients in finding ways to continue performing activities they had done previously and could no longer do. Or, if that was not an option, she might be able to help patients explore new hobbies.

She spent some time learning about my interests. She mentioned painting. I had always enjoyed arts and crafts, but I thought that I could no longer do them because of my arthritic, shaking, and uncoordinated hands. But Judy found a way for me to paint. She pulled out a stained-glass kit from the closet. The pattern was already fixed on the glass; all I had to do was fill in the colors. She wrapped a large piece of foam around the paintbrush to make it easier for me to grasp, then placed a quarter-pound weight around my wrist to steady my hand. I found the experience of painting both calming and exciting. With these adaptive tricks, I was able to paint again! When I came home, I proudly placed the glass oval, a picture of a covered bridge standing next to a pond, in my window where the sun streams through it.

After I finished in recreational therapy, I was sent to the psychologist, who met with every patient three times a week. I liked Eileen immediately and felt comfortable confiding in her. In fact, I felt at ease with all the therapists I had met. They were young, creative, dynamic people, mostly in their twenties and early thirties. I respected their knowledge and skill and responded to their warmth and caring. Each of my therapists' personalities and approaches was different, though the therapists all joined together to form a team that delivered me excellent, coordinated care. There was my physical therapist, Annie, soft-spoken and mild-mannered. She was so delicate and petite that I wondered how she worked with the many patients who were much larger than she. My occupational therapist, a young woman my age, was one of the bluntest and most direct people I ever met. The word "salty" comes to mind when I think of her personality. But Sam was as devoted to her patients as sweet Annie.

I was equally impressed with the doctor and resident assigned to me. I was introduced to Dr. Daniel, who specialized in neurologic rehabilitation, and her resident, Dr. Kramer, on that first full day of rehab. They were as compassionate as the rest of the staff. Both doctors, especially Dr. Daniel, who did most of the talking in that initial meeting and who conducted the examination, struck me as extremely intelligent, well-informed, and perceptive. When I spoke to Dr. Daniel, she listened and responded with thought and care. In her presence I felt the same safety and calm as with Dr. Marshall.

Everything proceeded smoothly until Thursday. That morning in PT, Annie and another therapist, Joe, approached me. Annie carried some kind of catalogue. They sat down beside me, and Annie said quietly, "We feel that you'd really benefit from getting a scooter. You're only walking eighty feet before you start to shake and have to sit down. The scooter would allow you independence. You could use the scooter for long distances and the walker for shorter distances." I looked at the pictures of the scooters and burst into tears. Dr. Machcinsky had mentioned the scooter, but I had never taken the idea seriously. With the force of a sudden gale wind, the realization that full recovery would not take just a few days of intensive rehab, and that my lifestyle at home might be changed, crashed into me. Joe put his hand on my shoulder while I pulled myself together. He eventually said, "No one is forcing you to do this. Just think about it." Annie had gone to bring me a glass of water and Kleenex. When she came back, she, too, said that the scooter was my decision. As she handed me the tissues, she said, "You know, it's O.K. to cry."

The afternoon unsettled me further. The social worker, Paul, who was a part of the rehab team, informed me that I was to be discharged on Friday or Saturday. The second insurance company refused to pay for more than five days. I felt furious that insurance was once again dictating the terms of my medical care. I did not feel ready to go home. What were the doctor's goals for me? What could I expect to be able to do when I was discharged? Obviously, their conceptions were different from mine. I felt confused and uncertain.

When Mom and Dad heard that I was to be discharged so quickly and the reason behind my speedy release, they were livid. They decided that BCBS was going to pay. My parents wanted to set their own precedent with BCBS, not allowing them to wriggle out of paying for the services our contract guaranteed. They decided on a new approach.

On Friday Mom contacted our congressman and senators and explained our dilemma. The congressman's office called BCBS and resolved the situation. The two senators' offices also called BCBS. The senior medical director of BCBS telephoned my parents personally to assure them that the company would pay for my entire hospital stay, which would last as long as my doctors felt necessary. The medical director swore that it had all been a misunderstanding. According to her records, I could walk 150 feet without any assistance. That was not the case, so BCBS would willingly pay. (My parents knew that there was no such record, but they had gotten what they wanted and decided not to debate the point.)

After my parents finished their conversation with the medical director, my mother asked my father, "Did she sound nervous to you?" My father answered, "Terrified!" Later that day, after the congressman had intervened, the senators' offices called my parents back to make sure that the problem was indeed solved. In a thick, gruff South Philadelphia accent, Dominick, a representative from one senator's office, said, "BCBS tells us that the problem's been solved. Is it true? We can't trust anything they have to say. Are you satisfied?" My parents assured them that they were. My parents received the distinct impression that Dominick broke legs and knuckles if his boss's constituents were not happy. If BCBS tried anything again, we decided, we'd unleash Dominick.

When I informed the social worker of BCBS's miraculous change of heart, he grinned. Paul said, "We can't tell our patients to do this, but your parents did the most effective thing they could. To keep the government from regulating their business, insurance companies pay large amounts to their lobby in Washington. They don't like it when congressmen and senators interfere in their affairs. They want the government to stay as far away from them as they can get."

Saturday arrived, and so did my friend Rachel, with whom I went to see, or tried at any rate, the Broadway show in December. While I was in the hospital, various friends from college visited me or called me. I was grateful for all of their support. But Rachel had to drive 150 miles from Maryland, and I appreciated that extra effort—especially after the disaster in December. I also enjoyed her slightly skewed sense of humor. She brought a card in which she wrote, "If you don't want the doctors to think you're crazy, stop answering the voices in your head!" In her get-well package, she included a video of *One Flew Over the Cuckoo's Nest*. When I pulled out a package of Reese's Pieces from the box, I was puzzled. She knew I could not eat them. But her card informed me that since these had worked for ET, she thought they might be useful to me. I should spread them around my room, and maybe my mother ship would come to take me home.

I used the weekend, with its far fewer therapy sessions and generally slower pace, to gather my strength. But at 3:30 Monday morning, I spiked a high fever, over 102°. Why can't emergencies occur at reasonable hours? After much blood was taken and various doctors were consulted, my physicians concluded that I had a sinus infection as well as some kind of upper respiratory bug. I was given antibiotics.

As part of the evaluation of my fever, I was sent down for a chest x-ray.

The transport person asked if I could hold my chart, which I did. He wheeled me down to x-ray and left me—and my chart—in the waiting area. I decided to make the most of the opportunity and read my file. There, on the admit slip to rehab, the first document the rehab doctors saw when I came onto their floor, was a long list of my diagnoses. "Lupus, lupus encephalopathy, pseudoseizures, thyroiditis, loss of appetite, weight loss. . . ." Pseudoseizures!

The diagnosis leapt out at me as if it were written in a darker ink than the others. Pseudoseizures, in the way that Dr. Gresley used the term, meant hysterical seizures. Her words from October came back to me. Her lie echoing through my mind. "The myoclonus looks atypical; it's probably coming from emotional repression. I can't speak about the cause or nature of the seizures, because I didn't see one. If you experience more seizures again, we'll retest and try to figure out what's happening." Obviously, she *did* make a diagnosis about the source of the seizures even though she never witnessed what my family and I called a seizure.

No wonder the doctors from the ER, physicians who did not know me, thought I was a nutcase. Dr. Gresley's summary letter from my October hospital stay was one of the more recent pieces of information in my chart. And Dr. Gresley was an extremely well-known and respected specialist in her field. Her label followed me and affected how others viewed me and my symptoms. My chart was poisoned by her diagnosis. I knew that I would have to deal with this issue at some point. I would discuss it with my doctors, especially Dr. Cohen. But the most pressing order of business was my recovery. I was now in the hands of capable physicians whom I trusted and who believed in the reality of my disease and symptoms. I would deal with Dr. Gresley and her diagnosis of pseudoseizures later.

On Tuesday Dr. Daniel came to my room for a visit. I brought up my concerns about going home. What were the goals rehab had set in order for me to be discharged? Not knowing what to expect when I got home made me feel uncertain and unsure. I knew I was supposed to go into outpatient PT after discharge from rehab. I had been to outpatient PT before. The program was wonderful and extremely beneficial. But my energy levels were so low that by the time I got myself to PT, I would be too tired to exercise. How would I be able to manage an outpatient PT program at this point?

Dr. Daniel replied. "How about we set up a team meeting with me, your physical and occupational therapists, your social worker, and the psychologist? Then we can talk about what we see happening when you go home and the expectations we have. You can ask whatever questions are on your mind, and we can all work on the issues together. Would your mom like to participate?" I replied that she would most definitely want to be there. "Could she be here by this afternoon?" Dr. Daniel asked. I knew my mom would make the time to come.

The entire group convened in a conference room. Speaking in turn, each therapist and the doctor used his or her own point of view to describe my major problems and how to deal with them. By this time I had adjusted to the idea of the scooter, which Sam brought into the room to show my mother. When faced with either staying trapped in my apartment, completely dependent on others, or making use of the scooter, I decided on the scooter. I chose to look upon it as something that represented freedom, not limitation. Besides, though rehab would take longer than I had anticipated, months instead of days, I did not view my current condition as permanent.

Both Sam and Annie emphasized that I needed to pace myself and conserve my energy. Both had noticed that I concentrated on finishing the task at hand and ignored my level of fatigue. They reminded me that I needed to stop when I grew tired, not when I finished whatever it was that I was doing. They felt secure that I would be able to handle living on my own. I could feed, bathe, and dress myself with the help of such devices as special silverware and a tub chair for the bathtub. I had been taught how to get up off the floor if I fell. In PT I had practiced walking up and down ramps and steps. Sam had worked with me on home safety, especially in the bathroom and kitchen. Paul gave me the number of a company that provided cleaning, shopping, and general services for the disabled; he thought that insurance might pay for some of it.

Eileen recommended that I visit Dr. Cohen after I left the hospital. "You've been through such a hard time, and Dr. Cohen provided you with emotional support you said you found helpful in the past." The psychologist and I also talked about my discussing the pseudoseizure label with Dr. Cohen. We hoped he would have some advice about how I could prevent that label from affecting my future care.

Last of all, Dr. Daniel reiterated the concept of listening to my body and not overdoing it. I asked what could be done about the spasticity, the severe stiffness, which was more prominent on my left side. When I walked, I dragged the left side after me like a piece of dead wood. As I covered more distance and became tired, the left arm and leg tightened and the hand curled into a rigid claw. It sometimes felt as if my entire left side would collapse out from under me. Dr. Daniel mentioned a new antispasticity drug. She had been trying to reach Dr. Fields in order to discuss that with him, but he had never returned her calls. She would continue calling him to ask about the drug.

After I was discharged, on Thursday or Friday, we decided, I would be followed as an outpatient by Dr. Daniel. She agreed that I would still be too weak to go directly to outpatient physical therapy, so I would be provided with home nursing, OT, and PT for a few weeks, until I regained enough strength to begin an outpatient PT program.

I left the meeting feeling greatly reassured. I knew what to expect. We had established a reasonable, realistic plan of action. Now I was emotionally ready to go back to my apartment. I began making plans for my return home.

The next day, on Wednesday morning, I waited in my room for my physical therapist to take me to the gym for therapy. As I sat in bed, I felt deeply chilled and had a headache. I walked to the bathroom and lost my balance on the way over. I kept myself from falling by grabbing the railing on my roommate's bed. Once I settled into my own bed again, I experienced some jerking and spasming of my limbs. I also felt nauseous. I thought, I must be spiking a fever again. I called for the nurse. She took my temperature, which was normal, and gave me the Tylenol I requested for the headache. I was not feeling well, but I went down to PT when Annie came to collect me. She started the session by having me do my exercises, which I performed on a raised mat.

She left me to my exercises while she attended to another patient. I began my leg lifts, but I felt increasingly strange. I do remember my entire body stiffening and jerking once and Annie coming over to me then dashing off. The rest has disappeared from my mind except for isolated images that float out of the blackness of memory; what I describe to you now I know mostly from what was told to me afterward.

Annie saw me convulsing, grabbed another PT to watch over me while she ran to find a doctor. Seconds later, Annie, Dr. Kramer, and Dr. Daniel rushed into the room. There was no doubt in either Dr. Daniel's or Dr. Kramer's mind: I was having a grand mal, tonic-clonic seizure.

I experienced several of these seizures, each lasting a few minutes. The color completely drained from my face, which had turned as white as the encased pillow beneath my head. The doctors hooked me up to a pulse-oxygen machine, which showed that the oxygen in my body had reached dangerously low levels. I had stopped breathing. I was put on oxygen, and I began breathing again on my own. Dr. Kramer tried to put in an IV line to administer an anticonvulsant, but he could not find the vein. These many weeks later, I still have a purple bruise the size of an egg. But I did not awaken or respond as he must have turned the needle this way and that, desperately searching for a vein as my body convulsed.

Dr. Kramer could not get a line in, but eventually the seizures stopped without medication. They brought my hospital bed down from my room and transferred me from the mat to the bed. This image comes vaguely to my mind, but the next thing I clearly recall is being in my hospital room, answering the nurse's questions. "My name is Melissa Goldstein. I'm at CGH. It's sometime in the morning, and your name is Lorraine," I replied. The docs and nurses were satisfied that I was now oriented as to time and place and had regained full consciousness. Apparently Dr. Daniel had asked me the same questions earlier. But that is gone from my memory. Dr. Daniel explained that gaps in memory are common after a seizure. Even after I came fully awake, I felt groggy and slow-witted.

After blood was taken, Dr. Daniel telephoned Dr. Fields to inform him of the seizures. She wanted to give me Dilantin, a general anticonvulsant effective for treating grand mal seizures. I currently was not on any anti-seizure medication; in October, Dr. Gresley removed my anticonvulsant, Depakote. I did not seize during the next few months. Depakote can be quite toxic, and apparently I did not need it on a regular basis, or so we thought. Though I knew Dr. Gresley stopped the medication because she thought I was a hysteric, I felt she made the right medical decision, even if for the wrong reason.

After speaking with Dr. Fields, Dr. Daniel came back to my room, per-plexed and distressed. Dr. Fields would not allow Dr. Daniel to give me the Dilantin. Dr. Fields stated unequivocally, "She's fooled us before. It's a pseudoseizure." Dr. Daniel argued with him, describing what she had seen, emphasizing that my oxygen level had plummeted and my pupils had shown evidence of seizure. She insisted that what she had witnessed were tonic-clonic, grand mal seizures, not pseudoseizures. Dr. Daniel had exten-sive training in neurology and was director of neurologic rehabilitation; she was perfectly qualified to diagnose a seizure. Also, she and her resident, Dr. Kramer, were the first doctors who actually saw the episodes that my family, nurses, and physical therapists thought were seizures. But Dr. Fields would not change his mind. He dismissed her knowledge, conclusions, and concerns as if she possessed the expertise of a first-year medical student. He did not come to see me himself, not then, and not later.

I was shocked, disappointed, and hurt by Dr. Fields's comment, attitude, and behavior. He did not say "it," when he referred to the disease, meaning that the lupus had fooled the doctors before. He used the pronoun "she," as if I had been intentionally manipulative or vindictive, producing the seizures for some bizarre reason of my own. To me, this was even more insulting than Dr. Gresley's diagnosis in which the pseudoseizures were seen as a form of true mental illness, something I was not engineering or faking.

Even if Dr. Fields did not think that I was consciously inducing my seizures, it was clear that he believed Dr. Gresley and her judgment of pseudoseizures. I thought that Dr. Cohen's psychiatric evaluation resolved that issue for him. Obviously not. During all those months, I had not realized that his perception of the seizures, my disease, and me had undergone a profound change. This doctor, on whom I depended, betrayed my trust in several ways. At the very least, I expected the truth from my physicians, even if I did not like what they had to say. I deserved at least that much respect. Dr. Fields did not even have the courage to tell me personally that he agreed with Dr. Gresley. He could not face me with honesty in October, and he could not do so now.

After Dr. Daniel communicated Dr. Fields's decision, she exclaimed, "How can I send you home without an anticonvulsant? Suppose you have a seizure while you're at home and don't come out of it on your own? The brain needs oxygen, and if you're deprived of it for too long, you can suffer from brain damage. You could fall and hurt yourself. I can't release you without some kind of seizure medicine. If you weren't already followed by neurology, I would prescribe it myself. But I'm not your neurologist."

Later that afternoon, I went for an EEG, a measure of brain waves. I do not know who ordered it. Dr. Daniel commented that the type of seizure I experienced came from electrical activity deep in the brain; an EEG would not be able to pick it up even while the seizure was taking place. Certainly, nothing would show up hours afterward. Knowing that this test was worthless, I could not wait to leave the EEG lab and return to rehab. I wanted to go for pet therapy, which was being offered that afternoon. Puppies and kittens were brought in for the patients to hold and watch. I thought that pet therapy was a much better use of my time than this test. Cuddling an animal would at least be soothing for the soul.

When Dr. Averapporti came in later, he overrode Dr. Fields's orders and prescribed Dilantin. This was no simple act. Overturning my regular neurologist's decision was an invasion of neurology's turf. But Dr. Averapporti's role as the physician who had coordinated my care for six years gave him some unofficial authority. This made his taking control of the situation less offensive than if Dr. Daniel, a newcomer to my case, had done the same thing. Still, Dr. Averapporti did not exactly endear himself to neurology, but my health, not his colleagues' egos, was his primary concern.

The next day, Dr. Daniel and I had a serious discussion about my neurologic care. She had again tried to convince Dr. Fields that I did indeed suffer from grand mal seizures, but he still did not believe her. I said, "It seems that I have this label of pseudoseizure, and he can't see beyond it. What should I do? Is there someone else in the neuro department that you work with and trust?" She spoke quietly, but firmly. "Melissa, you need a second opinion for your seizures. And you must go outside CGH to get it. Something like this gets very political. One CGH neurologist isn't going to contradict another." Though I appreciated her honesty, I could not believe a CGH doctor was telling me to leave the system, that I could not receive the care I needed at CGH.

Fortunately, my family knew a neurologist, Dr. David Lighton, an M.D., Ph.D., associate professor of medicine, and the director of a movement disorders clinic in a large teaching hospital also located in the city. He treated my great-uncle, my grandmother, and my mother. My family members, each of whom suffered from different neurologic disorders, were all impressed by Dr. Lighton's knowledge and his kindness. My mother left a message with his office. Without even knowing the reason behind the call, Dr. Lighton telephoned back within ten minutes. My mother gave him a brief account of my flare, our current dilemma, and a description of what Dr. Daniel had seen.

Dr. Lighton agreed that I had suffered a tonic-clonic seizure. My mother did not tell him about my aura before the seizure, but without her mentioning it, Dr. Lighton said, "I bet I can tell you what she experienced right before the seizure. She felt a profound temperature change. Either she became extremely hot or cold, and she had a headache. She might have been nauseous as well." My mother was shocked at his accuracy. He continued, "With these kind of seizures, she absolutely needs to be treated with an anticonvulsant. These seizures can be dangerous. And I want to see her independent and back to her usual routine; I don't want the seizures interfering with her recovery. She can't use the scooter if she is having seizures, and that scooter will really help her get around. I don't have privileges at CGH, but I can come to see Melissa on an unofficial basis. If CGH won't allow that, call me when she's discharged, and I'll see her in the next day or so. Have Dr. Daniel telephone me so that we can talk."

Mom and I both felt relieved. Though Dr. Daniel would not allow him to visit me on an unofficial basis while I was in the hospital, I would see him as soon as I was discharged. I also felt angry. For the past few years, I had told Dr. Fields, then more recently Dr. Gresley, about always feeling a terrible, sweeping sensation of coldness before a major seizure. Dr. Fields and Dr. Gresley had looked at me as if I possessed four heads. Yet apparently this was a textbook precursor for a grand mal seizure. What else had neurology missed? This hospital stay, and the visit to the epilepsy unit in October, did not inspire much confidence in CGH neurology's diagnostic skills.

Finally, two neurologists, still not Dr. Fields or Dr. Gresley, wandered down on Friday afternoon, three days after the seizures had taken place. They wanted me to come back to the epilepsy unit in order to monitor me on the EEG machine for seventy-two hours. Then they would decide if I really experienced seizures. I paused a moment, not sure how to phrase my answer. First I inquired, "Who would be in charge?" When I found out that it would be Dr. Gresley and a colleague, I hesitated again.

The neurologists noticed my definite lack of enthusiasm about my returning to the epilepsy unit and asked if there were some problem. In a calm, quiet tone, my voice firm and steady, I told them how I honestly felt. "I'm not comfortable with Dr. Gresley. I was extremely disappointed with her. Though she didn't witness a single episode which I or my family would call a seizure, she made a diagnosis of pseudoseizure. She then came up with a psychiatric explanation for these pseudoseizures—without consulting my psychiatrist, who has known me for the past several years. That's unprofessional as well as arrogant. Her diagnosis has stuck with me and seriously compromised my care.

"I've been through this so many times before. Doctors are faced with symptoms they can't explain. So they paste on a psychosomatic label, because they don't know what else to say. A few weeks or months later, the doctors find out what is really causing my medical problems. But in the meantime, I'm bounced to the psychiatrists, who declare that I'm perfectly healthy emotionally, and that my problems are not psychiatric. I then get tossed back to the medical people. I'm not a ping pong ball; I'm a human being. I'm tired of playing this game, and I won't do it anymore. None of this is directed at you personally, but you need to know where I'm coming from."

The neurologists faced me with expressions of stone and spoke not a word in reply to all that I said, except, "If you decide to come upstairs, tell

us by two o'clock." I followed up my refusal to be monitored by the epilep-
tologists with a letter that Mom hand delivered to Dr. Fields's office. I requested that a copy of my records be made available to me by the time I
was discharged. Because Dr. Gresley had so mismanaged my seizure diagnosis and treatment, I was seeking a second opinion for evaluation and
treatment of my seizures. He never responded to that letter either, though
a week after I was back in my apartment I received a copy of my neurologic
records. The envelope contained no personal letter of explanation or apol-
ogy. By this time I should not have expected anything, but it was hard for
me to let go of the image I had of Dr. Fields as the concerned, empathetic
neurologist who had cared for me these past five years. At least he was still
meticulous about his paperwork.

The weekend passed by uneventfully, though in some ways the quiet
fell with the force of a blow. Until this temporary hiatus in crises and major
decisions, I had no time to process anything. I was buffeted about by one
event after the other, but was too busy dealing with the practical matters at
hand to know how I *felt* about what was happening to me. I remember
being most distressed by the seizures themselves. I had been seizure-free
since September. When I experienced the aura this time, the thought of a
seizure did not even enter my mind. A part of me clearly believed that the
seizures, one of the most terrifying aspects of my disease, were gone—
permanently. They belonged to my past, like a particularly nasty nightmare
from childhood. But seizures and antiseizure medicines, with all their side
effects, were a part of my life once more.

I thought of the time before I flared in December. From the middle of
October through November was a period of calm for me, the lupus more in
control than it had been in years. Dr. Fields hoped that this improvement
signaled remission. No one had spoken that word to me in so long; in my
mind, it sparkled like a jewel, making promises of a rich, new life. I made
plans to begin teaching again. Then the disease cruelly snatched it all away.
So I grieved, not only for all that I went through these past few months—
the debilitating pain, the dependence on others, and the disappointments
in my hospital family—but also for the loss of the possibility that my turn
had finally come, that after nine years of unrelenting disease, remission
would be mine. I knew that this setback did not mean that I would never
go into remission. But the contrast between my expectations at the beginning of December and the present knifed through me, drawing bitter tears
instead of blood.

And the trauma of this hospital stay was not yet over. On Monday, I was scheduled for nerve conduction tests, which Dr. Averapporti ordered two weeks ago. I assumed that neurology would be conducting the tests; the neurologists had always performed these studies before. But I was slightly surprised. As I said to the resident when she came to inform me that I would soon be taken for the tests, "I'm surprised neurology's willing to do this. I thought I'd be unwelcome there."

The resident said flatly, "You are. Rehab medicine's conducting the test. We had grand rounds on Friday. Remember when we videotaped you walking and asked if we could present your case and the tape during rounds? Well, we had a number of suggestions and were concerned about your seizures. Neuro basically said that if we thought we knew how to treat you, then go right ahead. Then they discharged you from their service. You're no longer a patient there. We took over your neurologic care." I could not believe what I was hearing. I had ticked off individual doctors, even fired a few, but I had never alienated an entire department. When I had gathered my scattered wits enough to speak, I said, "You mean they threw a temper tantrum?" The resident nodded, "Yup."

It was the final betrayal. An entire department put ego ahead of my care. Neurology acted the part of a prima donna; if the neurologists could not occupy center stage, unquestioned and preeminent, they would play no role at all. May the patient be damned. Not one neurologist even showed me the courtesy or respect of speaking to me about their decision. Until the rehab resident informed me otherwise, I thought I still received my primary neurologic care from CGH neurology. Never, at any point, did I say, or intimate, that I was transferring my main neurologic care to another neurology department. When I wrote the letter to Dr. Fields stating that I would visit Dr. Lighton for a second opinion about my seizures, I made it clear that I was dismissing Dr. Gresley, but no one else. I never left neurology; the department abandoned me. Now there was a gaping hole in my health-care team. If neuro would not treat me, who would care for me if I were hospitalized again at CGH and needed neurologic treatment? Dr. Lighton did not have hospital privileges at CGH. What would I do?

Mostly, I felt hurt and bereft. My neurologist and the entire neuro department were an integral part of my hospital family. I was the darling of the department. I knew most of the residents and attendings. I joked, teased, and flirted with many of them. Each Christmas, I sent the department a package filled with cookies and candies. And Dr. Fields always received a

Christmas card from me in which I expressed gratitude for his wonderful care and my heart-felt wishes for a happy holiday and new year.

At least rehab, mainly Dr. Daniel, I suspect, took responsibility for my care. When the critical moment came, Dr. Daniel did not worry about whether or not it was politic to fight for her patient and contradict the neurologists' opinion. My welfare came first. I am grateful to her for that, and I think of her as another guardian angel who watched over me during this flare. Actually, when I look back to this hospital stay, I realize that, in losing one department, I gained another.

Tuesday morning was my date of discharge. Before I left, I was scheduled for an MRI of my brain and cervical spine. The test lasted about an hour and a half. While I was in the tunnel, I had time to think. There was a mirror directly above my head. The glass reflected the room outside in order to reduce the claustrophobic effect of the machine. As I looked up at the mirror, it became like a movie screen, and the events of the last few months, especially these past three and a half weeks in the hospital, replayed themselves.

As I watched the story unfold, I realized that I no longer considered CGH my family. That feeling of safety and protection within the hospital walls was gone. I understood then that no hospital could serve as a kind of family, providing that same sense of shelter and haven. I could trust and rely upon individuals, but not an entire institution. I had Dr. Averapporti, Dr. Daniel, Dr. Cohen, and many other health-care professionals along the way, during this flare and in my past, who had offered their competent care and kindness. I would have to accept that there were as many uncertainties in my medical care as there were in my disease. I would have to be ready to advocate for myself to ensure that I received the medical care I needed and deserved.

After the MRI I returned to my hospital room and, with my mother's help, packed my things. I wished everyone good-bye. Ten minutes after leaving the hospital, I found myself back in my apartment. Holding onto my walker, I roamed around my cozy home, through sight and touch reestablishing contact with my domain, leaving the hospital and the world of illness outside my front door. My hands drifted over the plush, pink velour of the recliner both sets of grandparents had given me as a birthday gift. I lingered over the many dolls from foreign countries, a doll collection gathered from my own as well as family's and friends' journeys. I noticed the smiles on the dolls' painted faces and caressed their silk, lace, and satin dresses. My eyes finally rested on my desk. There sat my manuscript, *Travels with the Wolf*, finished at the beginning of December, the crisp white pages stacked in a neat pile I had proudly made. I considered the manuscript for several minutes, thinking of all that I had written.

My mind filled with memories as I walked over to the window and gazed out to the river below. I had long been a river watcher. I had witnessed how it changed through the seasons, its banks overflowing after spring rains, the waters becoming a muddy brown as storms churned the river bottom. In summer, the river ran turgidly, slowly in the hot, thick air. In autumn and winter its blue waters sparkled under the cold sun. I have never seen the river freeze over; it seems determined to move forward as though pressed to arrive at its destination. But I did not know from where the river originated; I did not know from where it came. So even though I watched the river each season, I could not say I comprehended it, not fundamentally.

As I looked out the window, I was lulled and soothed by the sight of the river. Though the river lay beyond the glass, plaster, and concrete walls of my apartment, the river felt a part of me and my home. I have always needed to live by the water; my home would seem barren and incomplete without a river, ocean or even a stream near it.

Watching the river below, I recalled my travels over the past nine years. I fell into a half-sleep made of memory, blue water and tufted green banks. As I drifted, the scene seemed to shimmer and become transformed. I floated down to the ground, and I found myself once again in the desert, standing beside its river. I turned to my right and saw the road beside me, the path I had traveled for so long. I looked ahead, and the road continued to wind its way east, far into the distance, its end hidden from me. But it was the river now that drew my attention. As I listened to the music it created as it flowed, I realized that it was the river that gave life to all who dwelled in the desert. Yet I did not know the river. Like any river, to truly understand it, I had to follow it to its source. Then I would comprehend the river, the waters which had sustained me throughout my travels. Then I could understand the journey itself.

As the rush of the water, the river music, filled my ears, the desert landscape surrounding me began to fade, and as it disappeared, I was transported back to my apartment. Once more, I was standing in my place before the window. I paused a moment, thinking of the desert river. Then I walked over to my desk, settled myself in my chair, and turned to my manuscript. As I read and reflected, past and present merged, creating a deeper understanding of my path through the desert.

Putting pen to paper, I set forth on my journey once more, in the re-telling and remembering still searching for the desert's heart, the river's source. Faithful Reader, come with me. We will travel together, and perhaps we both shall find meaning and peace. So let us rest a moment, then continue on, back, back. . . .

PART II

SEPTEMBER 1969–PRESENT

4

The Mountain

September 1969–April 1988

OR YOU and I to understand my story, I must start with my growing up on the mountain of good health. When I look back to the time before I became sick and then to my illness experiences, I realize how deeply they are intertwined, that the first explains and gives context to the second. For it was on the mountain that my life took its shape. Illness never occurs in a vacuum; it assumes its form and meaning in the presence of a life, bounded and defined by an individual's personality, hopes, dreams, values, and relationships with others.

When I cast my mind back to my growing up, what comes to me most strongly are memories of family: my parents, Larry and Sandy Goldstein, and my brother, Jonathan, as well as my extended family consisting of both sets of grandparents, two sets of aunts and uncles, four first cousins, a host of second and third cousins, and great-aunts and uncles. I knew three of my great-grandparents.

It is my parents who come most vividly to my thoughts. It was as if while I grew up, through the accumulation of everything they had been, and done, and taught, my parents created diamonds, pearls, sapphires, emeralds, and other stones of beauty which they stitched with great care into the pockets of my being. And told me to remember what I carried. But when I left for college, like most young people I rushed forward into the beginning of my adult life, my hands open and reaching, searching to fill myself with everything that was new and of my own making, not understanding the value of all that I already possessed. But later, as I walked through the desert land, I jammed my angry fists into those pockets and rediscovered the beautiful stones that would now help me along my desert path.

Such as music to fight the physical pain of my disease. My earliest recollections are of my mother sitting on the edge of my bed and singing me to sleep as she accompanied herself on a classical guitar. Music is her way of celebrating, mourning, and thinking; I hear the speech of her soul when she sings and strums her guitar. When she sang to me, I heard her love for me in each note. Even now, when I hear a classical guitar being played, I feel a sense of well-being, as if the music is enfolding me like my mother's arms.

My brother's and my love for music, inherited from my mother, found expression first in the piano. Our lessons began when we were still small children. Today Jonathan is an accomplished pianist whose music brings him joy and solace. Later in elementary school, I also began flute and voice lessons. In high school, I sang in choirs and participated in musicals. Though my father played no instrument, he was always our appreciative audience.

The family life my parents created included both spontaneity and structure. Ours was a tumultuous, busy household, overflowing with people and animals. Both my parents worked partly from our house. The doorbell constantly rang as people associated with my father's business and students my mother tutored came and went. My mother bred dogs, samoyeds. In fact, my parents claim that their first child was Snowball, my older samoyed sister. At one point we also had a rabbit, a turtle, fish, and hermit crabs. My brother's and my friends looked forward to coming to our house. There was always something interesting going on there.

But despite the chaos, there were some rituals that gave pattern and form to our family life. No matter how frantic our schedules became, especially as my brother and I got older, the family ate dinner together. It was our time to find out what everyone had done during the day. It was also a time for learning and discussion. The topics ranged across the sciences and liberal arts—physics, computers, math, history, literature, and current events. When I was a young teenager, my father began a computer software business. Dad turned our basement into offices and worked from home. Often my father's computer programmers, my brother's friends, or my friends would join us. My mom's table was open to all.

Another ritual. Each day, when my brother and I returned home from school, we would go down to my father's study to let him know we were home, and we talked about our day. I do not remember my father ever asking us to do this; it came about naturally. I never knew how important this custom was to my father until one time when I neglected to observe it. He eventually came looking for me. He did not reproach me, but later my mother told me that my father had been hurt and had missed my usual afternoon hello. My father, though demonstrative and affectionate, does not communicate his deeper feelings with ease. My mother often acts as the go-between, saying what my father cannot. From then on, I never forgot to go down for our daily chat.

I recall, too, the holidays when the smells of good cooking wafted through the house, and the rooms rang with the laughter and conversation of relatives and the shouts of children at play. Summers brought vacations to the Maryland beaches. Often, the extended family would come too— aunts, uncles, cousins, and grandparents. From the beginning, I was fascinated by the ocean. I crowed with delight as I jumped the waves, exulting in the feeling of being lifted to the sky. I see my father, mother, brother, and me, our hands linked as we rode the waves together.

As memory and understanding merge, I realize that the most influential part of my growing up was that I came from a family of teachers. My mother has a master's degree in special education, and she worked with children and adults with learning disabilities. She performed testing and evaluations, tutored, and acted as an advocate in the school system, making sure that the learning-disabled child's educational needs were met. Like my father, she had her office in the basement. Every day I could see the effect she had on her students. Many of these people were extremely bright and gifted, but their disabilities prevented them from making full use of their talents. Often frustrated and ashamed, many of these students did not believe in themselves. But under my mother's care, her students gained confidence as well as skills and knowledge. I admired and respected her, and still do.

During most of my childhood, my father was a professor of mathematics at the University of Maryland. He was dedicated to his teaching and won several teaching awards over the years. I learned about the academic world through his experiences, and as I grew older, I came to want that lifestyle for myself. My mother often brought my brother and me to the university. The University of Maryland was originally an agricultural school. I looked forward to roaming the campus, with its large, green lawns and graceful, columned Southern colonial architecture.

We sometimes listened to my father lecture. I saw him at the podium speaking to hundreds of students. His face was animated and excited, for he was eager to share his knowledge. One day on campus a student rushed up to my father. She said, "Dr. Goldstein, you probably don't remember me, but I was in your math class a few years ago. I never understood math before you taught me. I can't thank you enough." I swelled with pride and thought "That's my father."

Some of my fondest memories are of the parties my parents gave for my dad's colleagues. There is one evening that I particularly remember. It was soon after Nixon had opened relations with China. My parents had invited a prominent Chinese mathematician to the party. He arrived along with a representative from the State Department, a secretary, and his own personal physician. The mathematician was a warm, grandfatherly gentleman, and I had quite a good time sitting on his knee listening to stories of his homeland. Many different accents could be heard that night—Russian, French, and British, to name a few. And music, always music. Many mathematicians, at least from what I have seen, are gifted musicians. And they filled my parents' parties with their music. Feeling secure and content, I would fall asleep to the sound of their conversation as well as the strains of the piano, the guitar, and voices raised in song.

These parties made me see that being an academic meant becoming part of a national and global as well as a local community, a perception reinforced by my father's travels. My mother, brother, and I often accompanied my father. My favorite trip was the summer we spent in Perugia, Italy, an ancient town famous for, among other things, its Perugina chocolates. I was about six and my brother four. During the week my father lectured at the university; on the weekends, we traveled around Italy. We visited Rome and Florence and ended the summer by spending a week in Lucerne, Switzerland. We took a train from Perugia through the Alps to Switzerland. We came upon Lucerne, and the lake for which the city is named, at night. I gazed in awe at the seemingly magical lake, which shimmered with starlight and the reflected lights of the town spread out on its shores.

Perhaps the most powerful recollection I have of my father's involvement with the academic world is his efforts to help a Russian Jewish mathematician leave the Soviet Union. I was in fifth grade at the time. The professor suffered from multiple sclerosis. He could not receive the kind of medical care he needed in the Soviet Union, but the government would not allow him to come to the United States, where he would be able to get proper attention. My father and other mathematicians at the university put pressure on the Soviet government, and the Russian professor, along with his family, was finally allowed out.

From watching my father, I learned that being a member of the academic world allowed one to reach out to others in a variety of ways. My father could affect the lives of his students, share knowledge and ideas with his colleagues, lend aid to others in need, and interact with people from diverse cultures and countries. My own interest in academia was a strong bond between my father and me. Years later, I understood how deeply that tie connected us. One afternoon, as I sat on a bench on the main path through the campus, I noticed a professor walking by,

> briefcase in one hand,
> child's hand in the other.
> Slowly they mount stone steps
> worn smooth by tramping feet.
> My mind fills with images of when
> my father brought me here,
> my small hand
> tucked securely in his.
>
> As we wandered through
> winding passageways,
> our footsteps echoed in
> long corridors haunted and heavy
> with learning gathered from the ages.
> This I sensed—
> but did not know,
> my chief delight being
> colorful, chalky clouds
> I created when I banged the erasers
> against my father's chalkboard.
>
> Now, the ivy walls have
> yielded up some of their
> mysteries to me.
> In tantalizing, urgent voices
> they whisper of many secrets
> yet untold.
> I open all my senses to
> catch their elusive siren song.
>
> The ponderous wooden door
> interrupts my reverie when it

makes a familiar creak
as man and child
enter the sanctuary.
I think they will pass by
without seeing me,
but, then,
as they cross the threshold,
he catches my eye.
In that moment,
father and son,
father and daughter
join in a coherent whole.
They all walk through together,
past and future merging
in their linked hands.

The ethic of helping others was one of the most important lessons my parents taught my brother and me, but I do not recall any specific lectures on the subject. Instead, my brother and I learned by their example, in the way they conducted their personal and professional lives. Like my father, my mother truly benefited people through her work. But from the time I can remember, she also took in what I thought of as the wounded birds, hoping to heal them with her care.

I particularly remember one young woman. My mother had stayed in the hospital for a few days. There she met Joan, her roommate. Joan had been in a serious car accident and had permanent liver damage as a result. She was a troubled person. She was about eighteen and had come from a poor, violent, and eventually broken home. She had little direction or support in her life, though she did mention that she might be interested in becoming a nurse. When my mom returned home from the hospital, she visited Joan often. While Joan was in the hospital, my mom held a family conference and asked us all how we would feel about Joan living with us. We came to a decision together; we wanted Joan to be with us. Joan stayed with us for a few weeks after she was discharged from the hospital but then she returned to her home in the south. We watched her leave with regret. I sometimes wonder what became of her. I know my mom sometimes thinks of Joan, too. But Joan's flight definitely did not deter Mom from taking others under her wing.

I see my mother in my brother. He too adopts those in need of his help.

When he was in elementary school, a friend's father died. Most of Jonathan's other friends abandoned this boy; they could not deal with death. My brother was very upset. He told my mother, "David is my friend, and I'm not going to leave him alone. I don't care what the others do." Jonathan kept his word. He and David are friends to this day.

My parents gave us a model of what it meant to lead a good life. They supported us in our interests. It was not important what career we chose to pursue, and as long as we could support ourselves, making a lot of money was not an issue. They wished for us to do our best and be happy with what we were doing. They wanted us to be independent, self-reliant, and self-sufficient, but they always made it clear that it was all right to ask for and receive help when we needed it. Most of all, a good life involved connecting oneself to others, in all kinds of ways, by offering one's concern, attention, time, and help.

The ethic of giving, of making a positive contribution to others' lives, was deeply instilled in me. It shaped me profoundly, defining what I wanted to be and do. This was one of the precious stones, a diamond, my parents sewed into the pockets of my soul. My legacy to carry with me. Later, unfortunately, it became a burden as well. For when I became chronically ill, the fear of only being able to take, not to give, devoured me, leaving a gaping hole which for so long I filled with shame and self-loathing.

My childhood, a time of health and strength, grows ever more idyllic in my memory, yet it was not perfect. Until I was about thirteen, I was extremely shy. I was outgoing with my family and my close circle of friends, but lacking confidence. I found it hard to make new friends. I was quiet and unsure of myself in large groups of people I did not know well.

Though I felt fairly secure about my general intelligence, my relative lack of aptitude in math upset me. Even more important, I was convinced that my appearance left much to be desired. I detested being plump and short. I hated my glasses. I was even dissatisfied with my curls, longing for thick, straight hair in a more exciting color than what I had decided was a rather ordinary shade of brown. My best friend in elementary school was everything I wanted to be—attractive, thin, certain of herself, smart (in math as well as in other subjects), and athletic. Though I was a good swimmer and liked to dance, I was terrible at team sports. Basketball, volleyball, kickball, and softball were the bane of my school existence. I used my weaknesses to measure my worth and found myself lacking.

My family constantly encouraged me, but my opinion of myself did not begin to change until about the eighth grade. At that time, I lost some weight, traded the glasses in for contact lenses, and met my first boyfriend. I remember him coming over to the house and handing me a note, telling me he thought that I was very pretty and nice, and if I would not mind, he would like to kiss me. I did not mind, and I received that first kiss underneath a maple tree in our backyard.

I concluded that I was not as ugly as I had thought. But that year, my self-conception underwent a more profound change than any improvement in my opinion about my looks could cause. The change actually began in fifth grade, when I wrote my first poem, the haiku about the eagle, and found that I could form a link with others through my writing.

In eighth grade, my interest in writing prompted me to take intensive writing seminars at Johns Hopkins University. Each Saturday my dad drove me to Baltimore for my writing class, which was part of an enrichment program for gifted and talented junior and high school students. "Writing Skills I—The Art of Rhetoric" consisted of a curriculum equivalent to a freshman college English course.

Every week we were given two essays written by two of our classmates. We had to write comments on their essays and be ready to discuss each person's piece during the next session. Each student was critiqued by the class twice every semester. It was during this year that I bloomed. I found the exchanges with my classmates invigorating. I learned how to give and accept praise and criticism, sorting out which comments were valuable to me. Most important, I began to have confidence in my skills. I would never be a mathematician, and I possessed no athletic prowess. But I had other gifts. I had words inside me and power to create beauty with them. I could reach out to others through the strength and clarity of my writing.

By the end of the year, I had been transformed. I was no longer the awkward, uncertain girl who had first entered the seminar room. On the last day, I gave my teacher a gift—a small box containing a seashell and a poem.

> I give to you this seashell,
> for it was my former home.
> Now I have relinquished it
> from its confines I have grown.
>
> I used to hide inside it,
> clinging to its security;
> too afraid to venture out,
> I hid from the world around me.

But I no longer need its shelter.
In the world I travel free,
So I give this in celebration
Of the person I can now be.

Over the years, my poetry became a conduit, a vital way to connect with others. When my great-grandmother died, I was thirteen. My family considered me too young to attend the funeral, so they made me wait at home. After everyone returned from services, I walked slowly down the stairs, afraid of the grief we all felt yet wishing to help in some way. When I heard my grandmother, Bubbe Leah, crying, I could not enter the kitchen. I crept back upstairs.

A few hours later, I returned with a poem about death as part of the cycle of living. My grandmother read the poem. Then we spoke about my great-grandmother, sharing our memories, telling well-worn, healing family stories and anecdotes. Later my grandmother told me how much comfort my poem had given her. She still has it, in a box with all my other poems, lovingly gathered over the years.

My writing, especially my poetry, also became a fundamental way for me to organize my thoughts, comprehend the life around me, and come to terms with my experiences. One early poem was inspired by my first visit to Philadelphia when I was about fourteen. On the way from Maryland, the train and then the bus passed through ghetto areas. I had been raised in the suburbs. Though my family and I had traveled extensively, we usually stayed in the tourist sections. In many ways I was still very sheltered and naive. I had never seen burned-out buildings and rubble-strewn lots. Even in the center of town, homeless people, often muttering in strange languages decipherable only to themselves, roamed the streets or slept on grates. People, some of them women with children, begged us for money. I was shocked and disturbed. Why did I have so much and they so little? Did I deserve my life? Had they done anything to merit their own fate? Were we really ruled only by random chance? The world no longer seemed so safe, certain, or just.

Whatever I came into contact with in my immediate environment, whatever events moved me or made me question myself or my world, became subject matter for my writing, particularly my poetry. My poetry began and has remained a poetry of experience.

I continued to hone my writing skills, for three years taking classes at Johns Hopkins. Then in the eleventh grade, I enrolled in regular

college English classes at the University of Maryland. By the time I left
for college, I realized that poetry would be my vocation.

> I glimpse a figure dressed in white,
> veiled bride covered in satin and lace.
> She shimmers with light but makes no sound.
> Silence surrounds her,
> but it is the stillness anticipating creation.
> I am afraid to approach her or gaze too closely,
> yet I cannot look away.
> Finally, she makes a gesture,
> I realize she holds a pen, her bridal bouquet.
> In fluid movement, she writes her message;
> it lingers in the air, a language of petals.
> She holds out her flowers and awaits my answer.
> Reaching toward her, I accept her blooms
> then gather my words, my wedding trousseau.
> I walk down the aisle,
> my bridal gown sewn in pearled poetry.

By the end of high school, the shy, timid little girl I had once been was
only a faint memory. A confident, outgoing young woman had taken her
place. I took great pleasure in my junior high and high school years, and I
especially enjoyed being at the University of Maryland. By my senior year
of high school, I was taking calculus and English classes at the university,
where I spent most of my time, studying and socializing.

It was in my math course that I met Carlos, my first love. He took me
to my prom and made it all that I hoped it would be. It was difficult leaving
him when it was time to depart for college. I was going to Laurel University
in Philadelphia, about a three-hour drive from my parents' house. I could
have stayed at the University of Maryland, but I felt that it was important
for me to go. I wanted the experience of living away from home. Also, by
this point, I was firmly committed to a career in academia. I planned to be
a scholar specializing in Victorian literature. I would teach, do research, and
write. Laurel had an excellent English department, and though my experiences at the University of Maryland had been extremely positive, I believed
I would receive a better education and be exposed to more opportunities at
Laurel. I was still so young. If Carlos and I were meant to stay together, our
relationship would survive the separation.

Though my parents would miss me, they were pleased and excited for me. Despite their feeling that the clock had ticked on too fast during my growing up, they knew that the time had come to let me go forward on my own. They sent me into my adult life secure in the trust, respect, and love that linked us. As for me, I looked ahead to my future with eagerness and anticipation. I saw limitless possibilities, if only I worked hard enough.

I was not disappointed. My freshman year was a time filled with the joys of exploration, intellectual stimulation, and emotional growth. The city swept me into its energetic, life-giving rhythms, so different from the sleepy Maryland suburbs where I had grown up. I made friends then who are an important part of my life still. These deep and enduring friendships were forged during late nights when we debated the major problems of the world, and solved them of course, cried together over crises of love and exams and celebrated all our various triumphs. When I returned home for vacations, I bubbled with news about my life at school.

But toward the end of my freshman year, in April, I became ill with a disease that did not reveal its identity until six months later. Chased by the beast of my illness, I tumbled down a rocky, unfamiliar path until I found myself in the desert of chronic illness. The land of good health, with its mountain and valleys was now barred to me. I stood in the desert, gazing up at the mountain, with its grassy, unreachable slopes. I searched for the green and gentle valleys, but in vain. Hidden from my sight, they lay some- where on the other side of the mountain.

5

Descent down the Mountain

April 1988–June 1988

W HEN I first began my descent down that rocky path, I did not see or anticipate the desert below. Like most young people, I considered my youth and usual vigorous good health an impenetrable shield that serious sickness would not penetrate. The valleys I had viewed from the mountain were still in sight, within my reach, or so I thought. For the illness came slowly, insidiously, masked as a mild nuisance. It was almost the end of the semester. Classes were in session, but final exams were fast approaching. I started to feel tired, but I dismissed this as end-of-term fatigue. When I ran low-grade fevers and experienced a general achiness, I assumed that I had some kind of virus. I was annoyed, not worried. I needed all my energy and concentration for finals. I did not have time to be sick.

I went about my usual routine, thinking that the symptoms would quickly disappear. But they did not. I remember sitting in astronomy class. We were learning about the geology of the planets, a subject I found extremely interesting. The professor was young and dynamic, and I looked forward to his lectures. But now I could barely stay awake; the effort was almost painful. I felt feverish and sluggish.

When Carlos and my parents heard that I was not feeling well, they insisted that I go over to Student Health. It was my first visit there. The doctor was a pleasant young woman who took my history, conducted an exam, and told me that she would draw blood for lab studies. She was concerned that I might have mono.

Mono! Catastrophe! I walked back up the street to my dorm with the word reverberating in my head. From what I had heard, it could take anywhere from a few weeks to a year to recover from this virus. For me, a person who had rarely been ill, weeks or months sounded like an endless amount of time to be sick. As I reached the dorm, I reassured myself, "Well, you don't know anything yet. It could still be some infection they can treat with antibiotics. It could go away before they even know what it is."

The doctor telephoned a few days later to tell me that I did not have mono. But I was dragging around campus, barely able to go to classes. I found it difficult to study. When Mom and Dad heard that I was still feeling sick and that the Student Health doctor did not know what was wrong, they said, "Melissa, we're coming up to Laurel and bringing you home, so we can take you to Dr. Katz." Dr. Katz was our family doctor who had been my physician from the time I was a young teenager.

I was not happy about the idea of going home before I finished the semester, but finals were still a few weeks away. I thought that I would go home, discover what was wrong, receive treatment, and return to campus in time to take my exams. Besides, my loving and concerned parents were not giving me much of a choice.

I returned to Maryland. It felt strange to be back again in the house where I had grown up. These past eight months, so many changes had taken place in my life. I walked into my bedroom. When I saw the dolls sitting on my hope chest and the miniature dollhouse tea set displayed on my bureau, I caught glimpses of the little girl from years past. I ran my fingers over the dolls' curls, their lacy dresses, smiled for the child I had been. But as I looked toward the books I had brought home, in order to prepare for exams, thoughts of the present and future filled my mind and heart. I realized for the first time that I had truly left home. Wherever my parents lived would always be a safe port of love, but it would never be my home as it was before. My home lay out there, wherever I would create it. I turned away from Raggedy Ann and the dollhouse tea set and immersed myself in the adult realms of philosophy, astronomy, Victorian literature, and American history.

Dr. Katz's first available appointment was not until a few days after I came home. During that time I developed abdominal pain on the lower right side. When Dr. Katz met with me and heard about the abdominal pain, he referred me, with almost no explanation, to a gynecologist. The gynecologist then informed me that Dr. Katz thought I might have a sexually transmitted disease (STD). If he had only asked me whether or not I was sexually active, Dr. Katz would have discovered that a STD was not a possibility. But Dr. Katz could not even broach the subject. I think that when Dr. Katz looked at me, he saw me as the child I had been when I first came to see him. He could not talk about sexually transmitted diseases with that child, so he avoided the issue by sending me to the gynecologist.

How differently I interact with my physicians today! Now I would never allow my primary physician to send me to a specialist without my fully understanding the reasons behind the referral. But in those early days of my illness, with passivity and blind trust, I placed myself in the doctors' hands. I had rarely visited physicians, so I drew my notions about them from books and the media, not from experience. American culture gave me my conception of physicians as wise, kindly authority figures who, with their possession of the mysterious and magnificent knowledge of Modern Medicine, occupied an almost omniscient position of power in a realm somewhere far above me. Therefore, I thought that all I had to do was present myself to be cured, and the doctor would make it so.

Naive? Inaccurate? Dangerous to me and unfair to my physicians? Yes. But in our society, this conception of the doctor as all-knowing angel is popular and widely held by laypeople as well as physicians. The opposite view is also propagated—the doctor as devil. But Satan was an angel before he fell from grace. Whether we perceive doctors as a group to be good or evil, many of us do tend to see them in terms of the divine. At least almost divinely powerful, if not divinely good.

The gynecologist had not provided any answers. We still did not know what was causing my symptoms, which fast were becoming worse. I looked anxiously at the calendar. I had arrived home a week before, and I had no answers, much less a treatment. Finals were almost upon me. I went back to Dr. Katz, who referred me to a surgeon. As I entered the surgeon's dimly lit waiting room, the first thing I noticed was a plaque that read, "Nobody wins in a malpractice suit." I was not encouraged.

The nurse ushered me back to the examining room and said the surgeon would be with me shortly. Meanwhile, I was told to disrobe and put on the by-now familiar paper gown, opening to the front. The gown was flimsy, short, and the paper ripped when I tried to tie the gown together.

I had felt embarrassed about exposing my body in such an intimate way with the gynecologist. After all, it was not as if I underwent frequent physical examinations; I was not even sexually experienced. But the gynecologist's gentleness clothed my nakedness and calmed my fears. In contrast, the surgeon's manner was abrupt and brusque. He seldom spoke except to bark out orders. He made little eye contact. To evaluate the abdominal pain, he demanded that I jump up and down and tell him if it hurt. This is no doubt a valid medical device to gather clinical information. But as I jumped up and down, clutching the bit of paper covering me and feeling like a performing animal, I felt incredibly embarrassed and humiliated.

The mind plays odd tricks sometimes, making memory conform to the associated emotions not the facts of an experience. I do clearly remember that, in addition to the paper gown, I was wearing short white socks, and my feet were extremely cold. I also seem to recall that I had been asked to take off all my own clothing except the socks. I know this must be false, since there would have been no reason for me to remove my bra and underwear. But when I think back to that visit, I do know that I felt overwhelmingly naked—stripped. That is the memory I carried away with me.

After conducting several unpleasant tests, the surgeon decided that I might have an unusual presentation of appendicitis, and that my appendix should be removed. At this point I realized that I would not be able to take my final exams. I contacted my professors and was given incompletes in my classes. My aunt Beth who lived in Philadelphia, her husband, and her children packed up my dorm room for me and stored my things in their basement. I viewed all of this as an irritating but temporary inconvenience. I would take my exams over the summer or in the fall when I returned to school. I was not overly worried about the surgery itself. Several friends of mine had undergone the same operation, and they had healed swiftly and without complications. After I recovered from the appendectomy, I would feel fine again. Life would go on as before.

I was operated on at my local community hospital. Because I was only eighteen, I was put in the children's ward. To my chagrin, I found myself in a room in which both walls and dividing curtains between beds were decorated with cartoon characters. I felt even more ridiculous when a volunteer offered me coloring books and video games.

During most of my medical visits, the doctors spoke mainly to my parents, not to me. When Dr. Katz called, if I picked up the phone, he asked to speak with my mother or father in order to discuss test results and what should be done next. Most of my early information about my illness was therefore secondhand. This frustrated me no end, but I did not fight against it then, for I thought this illness would be resolved soon. I did not consider it a threat to my way of life. Though most of me rebelled at the thought of being dismissed in such a way, demoted from young adult to child, I must admit that a small part of me found it comforting to be taken care of for the short time I would need until my life returned to normal.

Finally the day of my surgery arrived. A few hours before the operation, I crumbled. I panicked. How much pain would I be in after surgery? The surgeon was going to cut into me and remove an organ! Maybe it was routine for him, but not for me! Then the nurse came in with some medication, Valium and Demerol, to make me relax. I do not remember what happened later, but according to my family, I became extremely cheerful when the drugs took effect. In fact, I started telling jokes. My family said I was hilarious. They were laughing as the nurses rolled me away to surgery.

I was not laughing or feeling very cheerful after the appendectomy. My appendix proved to be healthy; apparently appendicitis was not my problem. I felt much worse after the surgery than before. The abdominal pain was excruciating. I continued to ache all over and run a low-grade fever. And I developed more symptoms. Within a few days after the surgery, my mother entered my room and exclaimed, "What's that on your arms?" I looked down to find that my forearms had become diffusely red. Also, I had always had rosy cheeks, but my cheeks had taken on a different, deeper red color that extended farther across and down than did my natural blush. Specialists from the infectious disease department were consulted, but they could find no evidence of an infection at work. Dr. Katz and his partner continued their investigations, though, as before, I knew only what my parents chose to tell me.

By this time I was becoming much more anxious. I still had no sense that I might have a chronic illness. But this sickness was no longer the irritating nuisance I had once thought. What could it possibly be? And how long would it take the doctors to discover the cause and, of most importance, cure it? Might it just go away on its own? I had plans for the summer. I was supposed to work in my father's software company and save money for college. I had invited a friend from Laurel, Teresa, to stay at my house for the summer while she worked for my dad. Teresa was from Jamaica and wanted to stay in the States for the summer. I wanted to do some creative writing, for it was difficult to find the time to write during the school year. My life was full; I had no room in it for sickness.

About two weeks after I was admitted to the hospital, I was finally released. April had blossomed into May. As I was wheeled out to the car, I gratefully inhaled the spring scents of flowers and cut grass, a refreshing change from the hospital smells. But as my mother drove out of the parking lot, she let slip the information that the doctors had repeatedly taken some blood test called an "ANA," which had consistently been positive. If I continued to run fevers and experience the other symptoms, then my doctor would refer me to a "rheumatologist." I had never even heard of such a specialist before.

There are certain moments in my illness that have stayed in my memory with the clarity of a living snapshot, complete with sounds, smells, tastes, and textures. I see my eighteen-year-old self sitting in the front seat, beige velour soft to my skin, a slightly musty odor in the car from when it was flooded during a hurricane the summer before. My mother has paused a moment in her departure from the parking lot. The expression on her face is one of guilt and defensiveness. She knows she should have told me before about the test and the rheumatologist. Teresa tries to make herself as inconspicuous as possible, pressing herself into a corner of the backseat. At first there is silence, complete, an emptiness which gradually fills with my fury, a fourth passenger in the car.

In later years, even as I fiercely guard and cherish my independence, I will understand and learn to have compassion for my parents' need to take care of and protect their sick "child." But at this moment, I do not care about my parents' needs or fears. With such pleasure and pride, I have just begun my life as a young adult. I will *not* go back into girlhood. I speak out of an anger fueled by the fear of what I might lose. "It's my life and my body. From now on, I expect you to tell me exactly what's going on." I glare at my mother, who snaps, "I was only trying to keep you from worrying. We don't know if you'll have to see a rheumatologist." I retort, "That's not the point. I'm not a child. Don't treat me like one." In a tight voice, my mother spits out, "Fine."

Over the next few years there were many such scenes between my parents and me—my need for independence clashing with their desire to shield me. For me, looking back nine years later, this moment marks the true beginning of my illness. As my mom, my friend, and I sat in the car, I still did not conceive of my symptoms as a potentially chronic, incurable problem. But in this argument with my mother, I began my fight to keep my independence and my identity. This struggle, more than any description of all my symptoms, is the story of my illness.

About a month passed. I healed from the appendectomy, but the low-grade fevers, rashes, nausea, aches, and extreme fatigue continued. I was not well enough to go to work at my father's company. Each day I watched Teresa leave for work. I felt ashamed and frustrated that I was not joining her. During the day, I tried to study for my exams. I would sit at my desk, my books in front of me, and I would find my eyes closing, as if lead weights pulled my eyelids down, down. Later in the month, I noticed that the joints in my fingers became red, swollen, and warm at times. I thought that I might feel better if I spent some time outside, enjoying the fresh air and sunshine. But I discovered that I had become sensitive to sunlight. Because of my fair complexion, I always had to be careful of the sun. This, however, was different. Not only did the rashes on my face and arms become worse when exposed to sunlight, but I also felt generally ill.

I called Dr. Katz to tell him what was happening. He referred me to a local rheumatologist, a type of doctor who specializes in diseases characterized by inflammation and pain in muscles or joints. By this time it was the beginning of June. As I sat in the waiting room, my hopes and fears mounted. Would I find answers here? Dr. Weissman took my history, ordered a large number of blood tests and referred me to a dermatologist.

I met with Dr. Weissman in two weeks' time to discuss the results. The dermatologist felt that the rashes were due to something called lupus. Based on my history, blood work, and a clinical examination, Dr. Weissman thought I suffered from either rheumatoid arthritis or systemic lupus erythematosus. He wanted to begin treatment with aspirin, but when I informed him I was violently allergic to aspirin, he gave me a prescription for a high dosage (60 mg daily) of prednisone, a cortisone drug. His discussion about the medication's side effects consisted of a warning not to eat too much because prednisone increases the appetite. He told me to return in a month for a follow-up visit and did not encourage me to call in between if I had questions or problems.

That was the last time I saw Dr. Weissman. He had not given me a definitive diagnosis. More important, he had not taken the time to talk with me and explain about rheumatoid arthritis (RA), lupus, or possible treatments. I was mainly familiar with arthritis as the aches and pains that people experienced as they became older. I had also heard of athletes developing arthritis. But how was rheumatoid arthritis related to these other forms of arthritis? If this was my problem, why had I become ill with it at that time? After all, I was only eighteen, and though I was physically active, I was no athlete. The other disease that he mentioned: lupus. I had never even heard of it. But I knew that lupus meant "wolf" in Latin. The fear of the unfamiliar combined with the rather gruesome name repelled me. Rheumatoid arthritis sounded much more benign. I thought. "If I have to have RA or lupus, please let it be RA."

When Dr. Weissman gave me the prescription for prednisone, I was stunned. I had heard enough about the drug to know that this high a dosage could wreak havoc on my system. Prednisone has many short- and long-term effects, ranging from mild to life-threatening. Since Dr. Weissman never explained at any length the nature of lupus or RA, his treatment plan seemed radical and unnecessary for the kind of symptoms I was experiencing. I wondered if there were other options besides prednisone or aspirin. Dr. Weissman's autocratic style, however, did not allow for questioning. Before I could gather my scattered thoughts and questions, his prescription was in my hand, and he was out the door. He had left me confused and frustrated. What was the real name of my illness? How should it be treated? By this point, I no longer accepted the doctors' opinions and advice with quite the passivity or blind faith that I had before. I threw away the prescription for prednisone and never saw Dr. Weissman again.

After I returned home from my visit with Dr. Weissman, my father looked up "systemic lupus erythematosus" in our Encyclopaedia Britannica's *Medical and Health Annual* for that year, 1988. My parents called me down from my room, with its stuffed animals, catalogues for the fall semester at Laurel, brochures for a junior year abroad in Paris, and the canopied bed where as I child, I had always fallen asleep as if I were sailing in a boat, floating safe and protected, into a sea of dreams. My parents handed me the article and waited quietly for me to finish.

In this entry, written in 1986, the authors define the disease as a chronic, inflammatory, autoimmune disorder that can attack anywhere in the body. Because lupus can affect any organ, any system, it can produce an astonishing array of symptoms. The disease can range from mild to fatal. It also has a pattern of exacerbation and remission. The diversity of symptoms and the pattern of flare then quiescence of disease activity makes lupus especially difficult to diagnose.

According to the article, about ten million people throughout the world are ill with lupus. Though I had never heard of it before, apparently it was not a rare disease. I learned that the majority of patients first become ill between the ages of thirteen and forty. More than 90 percent of these people are women. Though there are men who suffer from lupus, it has gained a reputation as a "women's disease."

The disease process stems from immune hyperactivity, but it is not known why the immune system turns on itself in this way. It appears that genetic and hormonal factors play significant roles in creating a predisposition to lupus. Various elements in the environment then act as triggers.

Possible triggers of the disease onset and flares include viral and bacterial infections; hormonal abnormalities; exposure to ultraviolet light; drugs or foods that increase immune function or decrease suppressor function; and genetic predisposition to hyperimmunity. The authors also state that the cause of abnormal antibody production varies in each patient.

As I read further, I became shocked at what I found. My own illness seemed to match the description given of systemic lupus. Though there is no definitive test, the American Rheumatism Association established a list of eleven criteria to diagnose lupus. In order for the physician to make the diagnosis of lupus, the patient should have at least four symptoms out of the eleven. And I did. My ANA test had repeatedly been positive (an indicator of an autoimmune problem), and I was experiencing photosensitivity, arthritis, and a malar rash (rash over the cheeks). Also, I was a young woman in my childbearing years, a member of the population most vulnerable to lupus.

Though the authors do discuss the worst-case scenarios of lupus and the treatments involved, their general tone is optimistic. They explain that even though lupus was once thought of as a rare, deadly disease, more often discovered at autopsy than in the doctor's office, today lupus is considered a chronic syndrome. For many lupus patients, the disease is mild and requires little to no treatment. Most patients suffer from moderate disease. Since the tenor of the article was generally positive, and I did not have any of the severe symptoms listed in the article, my shock and surprise came not from fear but from recognition. I saw how my illness over the past summer could be attributed to this disease.

I needed to find another rheumatologist. If we could just identify my illness, whether it was lupus or something else, I could begin treatment and resume my normal routine. My brother's internist/allergist suggested that I consult with Dr. Smith, a rheumatologist at one of the most prestigious university hospitals in the country. The earliest appointment available was at the beginning of August. Despite the wait, my parents and I eagerly made the appointment. After all, she was noted in her field of rheumatology, and she was a specialist in lupus. She would be able to solve the riddle, put a name to this illness, and restore me to my usual healthy self.

6

Wandering in an Unnamed Land

June 1988–August 1988

I PASSED the next month and a half as I had the many weeks before, feeling as if I were in a state of suspended animation. In fact, when I think back to those pre-diagnosis months, it is the continual waiting that I remember most—waiting in the doctor's offices and laboratories, waiting for the doctor to call back with test results, waiting for explanations, but most of all waiting, sure (at least almost certain) that the symptoms would recede and normalcy would soon return.

I tried to put my health problems aside. I struggled to study for my final exams. Whenever I could, which was not often, I went into work. I spent some time with Teresa and my friends from high school. Through telephone conversations and letters, I kept in touch with my newly found college friends. But I found that contact with my friends often proved awkward.

I clearly remember my friends from high school and me getting together for a summer reunion. Six of us met at Jill's parents' house for a barbecue. Before eating, we all sat in Jill's living room. We formed a circle, and each person took a turn talking about life in the first year of college.

I spoke enthusiastically about Laurel—my friends, classes, plans for the future. But while I was describing my life at school, I felt as if there were three Melissas in the room—the friend from high school, the young woman in college, and the ill Melissa. I did not know what to do with that third Melissa. She did not feel like a part of me; she seemed more like an unwelcome stranger who had chosen to visit. She did not occupy a welcome place in my own head, and she definitely did not fit in here with these glowingly fit and healthy young women who had no experience of prolonged or serious illness. I tried to cut my narrative short and not mention the summer. When Jill pressed me, I just said that I was working in my dad's company part time while I was recovering from having my appendix taken out. I was asked no further questions about my summer activities, but as they all described their jobs and vacations, I felt very much ashamed of my lack of productivity and resentful of the time lost to me.

During that summer, and throughout my illness, fatigue was, and would continue to be, the most overwhelming problem. It was worse than the pain. It was not the same tired feeling I used to experience at the end of a busy day or because I had not slept enough. This fatigue clung to me from the moment I awoke, even after I had slept around the clock, and became worse as the day wore on, each small task becoming a seemingly insurmountable obstacle. I was so exhausted that it became increasingly difficult to work, study, or go out with my friends.

> There are two fiends who come knocking at my door;
> Though I beg them to visit me no more,
> They ignore all my entreaties and pleas
> Saying I will have their company.
>
> In anger and fear, I fasten the locks,
> But my show of strength they mock.
> Suddenly by my side they appear;
> Their faces are so loathsome and drear!
>
> The one dressed in crimson calls himself Pain;
> Fatigue wearing black is the other one's name.
> Though Pain's blazing fire I detest,
> Of the two companions, I mind him less.
>
> Fatigue's evil is more odious to me;
> His blackness swallows my bright energy.
> Gone are love and laughter and hope
> While through the void of apathy I grope.
>
> Pain with his friend to instigate
> Frolics through me at a furious rate.
> Pain's presence is so much harder to bear
> When Fatigue accompanies him—a hateful pair!

So if I must let these devils in my door,
To these despicable foes I do implore,
"Let your visits be very far and few.
Fatigue come not. Pain is more welcome than you!"

During the day, while I was occupied, I could keep my fears and anxieties from rising to the surface, but before I went to sleep, out of the depths
the worries would emerge and run through my mind like evil imps. Surely
this rheumatologist would be able to help me. But time was passing so
quickly, and so much of the summer had already been lost. As I lay awake,
I thought about my life at Laurel. My classes were important to me, but so
was my social life. I greatly enjoyed living at Washington House—a dorm
and a special university program that sponsored a variety of events. Faculty
and their families, graduate students and undergraduates, formed this community, of which I had become an active member. I had also joined an
English honor society that had its own full calendar. I frequently went out,
especially dancing, with my friends. College was all I had dreamed it would
be. But it took energy and strength to maintain that kind of hectic schedule.
Would I be back on my feet again by September? Would the doctor resolve
my symptoms in time for me to start school and continue as I had before?

I would drift into an uneasy sleep. Day would return again. Though
discomfort and fear were always present, I also remember jokes and laughter. My mother always told me that my sense of humor was one of my
strengths, and I used it now to make the situation bearable—for myself
and others. It was particularly helpful when I discussed my health problems with my friends. Eighteen- and nineteen-year-olds do not usually have
much experience with illness. My friends wanted to be supportive, but they
did not know what to say or do. I did not want to burden them or scare
them away, so I relayed information about my health through humor.
When I spoke about the latest x-ray or other test involving radiation, I
would quip, "My parents have sold the microwave. I just breathe on the
food, and it's done in a minute!" The diagnosis that the doctors wrote on
their billing sheets was "FUO," fever of unknown origin. I told everyone
that the doctors had labeled me a UFO, unidentified feverish object.

I was trying to lighten the mood with my humor, yet some of my true
feelings were buried beneath the jokes. Sometimes I truly felt as if I were an
"unidentified feverish object." Certainly many doctors made me feel like
an object instead of a person. As a result of the way they interacted with

me—as well as the illness itself, which was preventing me from working, writing, studying, and socializing the way I usually did—I sometimes felt as if I were becoming unidentified, somehow losing my usual self. That sense of being unidentified and dislocated was heightened by not knowing what was wrong with me.

During these months I spent as much time as I could in the familiar world of books and writing. It was not a time of writing poetry, but I did keep a journal. I turned to books, particularly novels, for solace and escape.

A friend of mine who knows my love for books and has a penchant for giving advice, as most people do on the subject of illness, gave me copies of Dr. Bernie Siegel's *Love, Medicine and Miracles: Lessons Learned about Self-Healing from a Surgeon's Experience with Exceptional Patients* and Norman Cousins's *Anatomy of an Illness As Perceived by the Patient: Reflections on Healing and Regeneration.*

Bernie Siegel discusses the power of the mind to heal the body. In other words, if you heal your life by improving your attitude, resolving conflicts, and letting go of anger and bitterness, then you can heal your body. In his view, illness stems from negative, usually repressed, emotions and emotionally unhealthy lifestyles. Siegel focuses particularly on cancer, but he applies the concept to all major illnesses. Norman Cousins tells the tale of his own illness. He states that through the power of positive thinking, in this case laughter, and high doses of IV vitamins, he was able to galvanize his immune system and cure himself of a life-threatening disease.

I had heard of both books before. They had gained widespread public attention when they were first published. *Love, Medicine and Miracles* and *Anatomy of an Illness* appeared in 1986 and 1979, respectively, and both are still in print. If one wanders into any major bookstore, they can usually be found on the shelves in the health section. As the front cover proudly proclaims, *Love, Medicine and Miracles* is a #1 *New York Times* bestseller and has now sold more than two million copies.

In these books I found a reflection of our society's beliefs about life-threatening and chronic illness. Over the years I have frequently encountered these notions about illness. These ideas about chronic illness are a double-edged sword. On the one hand, the idea that this collection of symptoms, whatever name we ultimately gave it, could be eliminated or at least controlled by my exerting some mental effort was enormously exciting. It gave the power over my future back to me. On the other hand, the illness beliefs that Cousins's and Siegel's writings represent placed the weight of cause and cure squarely on my shoulders.

This was a heavy burden to bear. Apparently other ill individuals were also troubled by Siegel's philosophy and advice. Despite the success of his book and its sequel, *Peace, Love and Healing* (1989), many patients wrote to him in anger, telling him that they did not appreciate being blamed for their disease. In 1990, he responded to these accusations in the introduction to his reissue of *Love, Medicine and Miracles*. He stated that he did not write his book to make anyone feel guilty; he only wanted to help people gain access to their self-healing power. Why do some people think that Siegel is blaming them for their disease? Siegel gives the following explanation: "What they are doing is seeing what they bring to the situation. We all project our problems and create our own metaphors. Just as disease can be used to heal a life, so can this book. If you find it inspiring, you are inspired and if you feel guilt, fault or blame please ask yourself where in your life experience did these feelings originate. This will help you to find the ability to love yourself and heal your life." The victims of illness are blamed again as Siegel tells his readers that any feelings of guilt are their own fault.

I wish that I had known in that summer of 1988 that others had reacted to Siegel's works as I did, for I felt alone with my guilt and shame. As I struggled with the uncertainty of not having a diagnosis or a treatment, I turned to books for illumination. There were no peers I could consult. I found no accounts written by other young adults going through experiences similar to mine. So I read books by Siegel, Cousins, and others of their ilk. These authors made me question whether or not I was causing my somatic disease by emotional ill-health. Yet I thought I had been happy and relatively well-adjusted. Could I have been so wrong about myself? As I turned these questions over in my mind, the thought of mental rather than physical illness as the cause of my symptoms made me feel a particular fear. This dread stemmed from the social stigma that is unfortunately and unfairly still often attached to mental illness. If mental illness was my problem, how could I tell my friends and family?

While I puzzled over my strange illness, my family did the same. Like me, they were confused by my mysterious illness; they were uncertain and afraid and wanted answers and reassurance. They were also very free with suggestions and advice. Shyness and timidity are not common in my family. When I would return home from a doctor's appointment, or my parents and I would receive news of test results, calls would go out to the relatives. Everyone had an opinion. Though I knew that their comments came from love and concern, their input sometimes made my situation more difficult and painful by exacerbating my own self-doubts and guilt.

My grandparents, Bubbe Pearl and Zaide, had a particularly hard time dealing with my illness. They were struggling with the indignities of aging, and they remembered their youth as the golden years of strength and health. So many times I heard them say, "Oh, but when I was young," and they would smile, caught in the bittersweet joy of reminiscence. They recalled their youth when their lives stretched before them, years of bright possibility, and old age was so remote, hidden in the mists of the future. My grandmother did not believe I could be suffering from arthritis or lack of energy at eighteen. It was not natural. My having a serious, lingering physical illness seemed unlikely to my grandmother, and in her love for me, she was hoping that I just had the blues or even a more serious case of depression. In her view depression was relatively harmless. It was something I could make go away if only I would adopt the right attitude. My grandmother continually asked my mother if I were upset about anything. My grandmother would tell me that I should get out into the sun, get some exercise, and I would feel better. I should also try to make it into work more often. She would say, "Too much lying about can make you feel sluggish, you know."

I did not really know how my grandfather felt. He is like my father, his son; he does not reveal his deeper emotions easily. I love both my grandparents; I respect them and the life they have made together. Whenever I envision how I want my marriage to be, I think of them. Even after more than fifty years of marriage, they still look at each other with passion. My grandfather's eyes still see the young woman he courted and married. They are friends, companions, partners, and lovers. I would count myself blessed indeed to find a husband like my grandfather.

My grandparents' good opinion meant a great deal to me. I could not bear the thought of them believing that I was a malingerer. I wanted them to know that I was not depressed, either. I would try to tell them about my encompassing fatigue, fevers, and pain, and that my "lying about" was not by choice. But whenever I tried to talk to my grandparents about my symptoms or visits to the doctor, they hurried off the telephone. I learned to talk about other subjects with them. But their comments, well-intentioned as they were, stung. I experienced the hurt that can come of love and concern.

In the middle of June, after making the appointment with Dr. Smith, my family and I decided that we all deserved a vacation at our beach condominium on the Delaware shore. Teresa stayed behind to work and came to the beach on weekends. Before leaving I met with Carlos. For the last time. From the beginning there had been underlying tensions in the relationship. He was well-educated and was studying for his master's degree in information systems management, but our backgrounds were different. He came from a poor family; my family was upper-middle class. I went away to Laurel; he stayed at home to study at the local university. I never cared about these differences. I loved him and respected him, and that was all that mattered to me.

But these differences in our backgrounds did matter to Carlos and were a continual source of irritation. He felt insecure about his family and his relative lack of wealth. He continually told me that he might never make a lot of money like my father. I tried to reassure him that becoming rich was not important to me. I certainly did not measure someone's worth or value by how much money he or she made. But I do not think he ever truly believed me. Throughout my freshman year at Laurel, the tensions between us escalated.

My illness finally severed the relationship. I felt that Carlos was not being supportive; he felt that I was not showing enough sympathy for him. In his view, he was studying long hours for his summer-school courses while I was taking it easy, being waited on hand and foot like a princess. Though our quarrels seemed to be about my illness, they were also fueled by the other stresses tearing at our relationship. He called once while I was at the beach, but we fought and hung up on each other. We never spoke again. Though the ending was not without pain, it was not unexpected, because we had been pulling away from each other for several months. By this time, I was ready for the relationship to be over.

While at the beach, I tried to let body and soul mend. I appreciated the hiatus from the doctors' appointments and medical tests. I took great pleasure in the sea, and I spent peaceful evenings out on the balcony letting the susurration of the waves wash over me, through me, and back out again, emptying me of all thought, letting all that was of illness wash out to sea. In this pleasant state, I drifted unencumbered, a part of the vast, clear nights. Though this was but temporary relief. My illness always waited on the other side of the sliding glass door.

Finally came the day of my appointment with Dr. Smith. As my mother and I got ready to leave, my father wished us good luck. He hugged me and called me his "Cookie," a nickname from my childhood, when my hero was *Sesame Street*'s Cookie Monster. Though he could not directly say it, I knew he was as worried and hopeful as my mother and I. We were all concerned, but we thought that day's visit would mark the end of this summer's sickness. I would be given a name for my illness and treated. I was going to one of the most elite hospitals in the country, where I would find the best that modern medicine had to offer.

As was his usual practice, my father did not accompany us to the doctor's office. When we arrived home, my father, anxiously waiting, would be given the news. This arrangement was partly a result of my mom's schedule, which was more flexible than my father's. His business required his presence during the entire workday, but my mother could adjust her appointments to tutor her students. Also, though my mother had a full-time career, my father was the primary financial support.

But the reasons behind my mother's going with me to doctors' offices were more than just practical. She had the emotional strength to cope with these visits and all their implications. We might do our best not to acknowledge it to each other or even to ourselves, but visiting doctors was an emotionally draining experience. It brought to the forefront all our fears about my mysterious health problems. What was really causing my symptoms? Would the illness get worse? Was it treatable? What did the treatment involve? My mother acted as a buffer, my father's protector.

About forty minutes after leaving the house, we arrived at the large university hospital, which was located in the worst part of the city. After circling the block a few times, we eventually found the garage and parked the car. The next challenge involved negotiating the maze of corridors in our quest to find the rheumatology department. When we finally found the office, I was surprised to find a spacious and luxurious waiting area. The plush chairs were of various pastel shades that matched the colors in the large, precisely hung paintings. The walls looked as if they had been freshly painted. In the center of the room was a huge tank filled with exotic tropical fish.

Despite the decor, the experience of being a patient there was like being processed through a ruthlessly efficient assembly line. As I entered the office, there was one small registration area. After I finished filling out forms, I was pointed toward the chairs arranged around the fish tank. Not long after, a nurse called my name and took me back to a little cubicle where she took my vital signs. Though not rude, she was not friendly either. Not a motion or word was wasted, and with the efficiency and speed of a machine, she ushered me back to the waiting room. After I waited another ten minutes or so, at exactly the time of my appointment, the nurse announced my name once again to escort me back to the examining room. She asked me to put on the gown she laid out on the table.

My mom stayed in the waiting area. Over the months, I had become much more assertive about my medical care. I did not want to be treated as a child by my parents or my physicians. My mom and I had worked out a compromise. Initially I spoke to the doctor alone; then, at the end of the visit, when he or she talked about his or her findings and opinions, my mom would join us.

Because of the elegant waiting area, I expected large, sumptuous examining rooms, but they were small and utilitarian, with just enough space for patient and physician. There were no decorations or personal items. I felt even more intensely that I was caught on an assembly line. All the discussions with Dr. Smith were conducted in one of these examining rooms.

Dr. Smith briskly entered the room. I had sent my medical records, so she knew most of my medical history already. After taking my history once again, she examined me, then asked a nurse to bring my mother into the room. Dr. Smith said that she needed to take extensive blood work to confirm the diagnosis and that she wanted me to consult with a dermatologist at the hospital. She felt strongly, however, that I had lupus, a mild case, which did not require cortisone therapy at that time. (Medically defined, a mild form of the disease is one that does not affect any major organs.) She had decided to use Plaquenil for treatment. This drug, an antimalarial, is much safer than cortisone and can be quite effective at controlling the rashes, arthritis, and fatigue of lupus. Dr. Smith stressed that people with lupus can live a normal life and even have children. She also made a diagnosis of what she termed fibrositis, but is now known as fibromyalgia, a chronic, noninflammatory syndrome of pain in the ligaments, tendons, and muscles. She emphasized the importance of exercise in treating fibromyalgia; she heartily approved of the swimming regimen I had already instituted for myself.

About a week later, Dr. Smith called me to give me the results of the blood work. Again there were no abnormalities except for the elevated sedimentation rate (a general indicator of inflammation) and a weakly positive ANA test. (The ANA tests performed over the past few months had been much more strongly positive.) She said that we would have to wait for the dermatologist's report on my malar rash to decide whether or not I had an autoimmune disease. Meanwhile, she knew that I definitely suffered from fibrositis and that I should continue my exercise regimen.

I then tried to make her understand my frustrations about not being able to work over the summer and my worries about not having enough energy and strength to keep up a busy schedule in the fall. She was my physician. I thought that meant I could confide in her. There was an empty pause before she answered. Then she coldly informed me that my inactivity resulted from excessive anxiety, not disease, and that there was no reason to be concerned about returning to school. She suggested counseling to help me deal with my anxieties. Either I could find someone on my own, or she could recommend the behavior modification unit at the university hospital. I was stunned. Before I could respond, I heard the click of the receiver, then the dial tone. She had hung up. And left me alone on the other end of the line.

When I told my parents what Dr. Smith had said, they, too, were shocked, disappointed, and upset. I was scheduled to see the dermatologist in a week; after that, I was supposed to go back to Dr. Smith. We decided to keep the appointment with the dermatologist and Dr. Smith. Perhaps the dermatologist could provide some answers. Maybe this was just some gross misunderstanding that Dr. Smith and I could resolve.

After visiting the dermatologist, I returned to Dr. Smith. I followed my usual routine, going into the examining room while Mom stayed in the waiting area. Dr. Smith began by declaring that the dermatologist had said that the rash was not caused by lupus; therefore, my only physical problem was fibrositis. Fibrositis is severely aggravated by psychological stress, so it was essential for me to learn how to manage my anxieties.

I tried to open the lines of communication between us by being honest about what I felt and thought. I was not hostile or confrontational. I was not meek in my tone or attitude, but neither was my voice raised or even aggressive. I said calmly, "Dr. Smith, I was really hurt by your comments over the phone the last time we spoke. I opened up to you, and I feel I only got slapped in the face for it. Also, your diagnosis of fibrositis as the only cause of my symptoms doesn't make sense to me. Even if we assume that the rash isn't due to lupus, a diagnosis of fibrositis still doesn't explain the elevated sedimentation rate or fevers which are signs of inflammation. Fibrositis isn't an inflammatory disorder. Fibrositis doesn't cause photosensitivity either. And even though the one ANA test you performed was only weakly positive, with a reading sometimes seen in 'normals,' all the ANA tests taken over the past four months have been consistently, strongly positive. Isn't it more logical to look at all the ANA tests as a whole instead of relying on one reading?"

I was trying to work out our personal differences and discuss my medical situation in a reasonable, analytical way. But Dr. Smith became livid. I had crossed a boundary by challenging her authority. I was a patient, and a relatively young one at that. My role was to listen and submit. When I asked if she would just speak to my mother for a few minutes, Dr. Smith refused. She stood up, pulled the door open, then spat out, "Our time is up."

After leaving Dr. Smith's office, I felt angry, bewildered, and frightened. The expert upon whom I had depended to unravel the knot of my health problems had given a diagnosis that made no sense to me. And she had told me in no uncertain terms—whatever the diagnosis, what I really needed was counseling to deal with my "excessive anxiety," which was exacerbating or even causing my physical symptoms. I felt as if my character had been attacked. I was already feeling guilt, shame, and self-doubt from my readings of Siegel, Cousins, and company. Commentary from well-meaning family members did not always help. Was I really suffering from a form of depression? Was I just warped, anxious, or plain crazy?

Dr. Smith's reaction had shaken me deeply. It changed the way I interacted with doctors. I decided that I should keep my emotions to myself when dealing with physicians; it was too dangerous to make myself vulnerable to them. I should relate my symptoms in as objective terms as possible and keep my inner self hidden.

My experiences with Dr. Smith shattered that innocent and naive view of physicians as uniformly kind, wise demigods or angels, far removed from me in skills and knowledge. I had learned that even though doctors were skilled and trained in ways that I was not, I possessed my own special knowledge—of myself and my body. I was able to think and reason. I needed to use my self-knowledge, as well as my powers of analysis, to decide whether or not a particular diagnosis or piece of advice made sense. I had to find a physician who would be willing to become my partner, a doctor who respected and was not threatened or offended by the contribution I could and must make to my care.

I could not believe that I had been ill for almost five months and yet still had no convincing diagnosis. Though these months seemed interminable, I later discovered that the average time between the onset of symptoms and the diagnosis of lupus is three years. I could only imagine how a person with undiagnosed lupus feels after years of looking for a diagnosis, perhaps having lost faith in him or herself and maybe even credibility with friends and family.

Over the next few years following my experiences with Dr. Smith, on an intellectual level, I came to better understand some of the forces that shaped our encounters. First, diagnosing lupus is genuinely problematic. There is no definitive test for the disease; the diagnosis is based on criteria set by the American Rheumatism Association. To further complicate matters, early symptoms can be vague and unspecific, waxing and waning over hours, days, months, or years. Often standard diagnostic tests do not uncover any abnormalities. The ANA test, the most sensitive and specific for lupus, can remain negative for several years after the onset of disease. And lupus patients tend to look wonderful even while feeling sick.

For these reasons, lupus is difficult to diagnose, but this does not fully explain Dr. Smith's behavior. A physician wants to fulfill his or her primary function of diagnosis and treatment, but in lupus, the main source of information often lies in the subjective words of patients instead of in laboratory tests that measure disease in terms of specific biochemical processes. The modern physician has been trained to rely upon laboratory data and "objective" evidence in the assessment and treatment of disease. Therefore, lupus, which often cannot be diagnosed or followed by using hard data as a sole or even primary source, can challenge the way in which the modern physician has been taught to approach the task of analyzing, explaining, and treating disease. This can cause friction between doctor and patient as the doctor experiences mounting frustration.

Frustration fueled Dr. Smith's reaction to me. Dr. Smith had almost made the diagnosis of lupus based on my previous lab work, history, and clinical examination and was even thinking of a possible treatment. But the results of the blood tests she conducted were not what she expected. When the blood work showed few abnormalities, she became unsure of her original hypothesis. My subjective symptoms and her own conclusions were not rendered into as objective terms as she would have liked. What had originally seemed almost black and white, faded into gray. Faced with uncertainty, she lashed out at me. She did diagnose me as having a somatic disorder, fibrositis, but she blamed me for it by telling me that my anxieties were a major cause of the disorder and its associated symptoms. As I later learned from my own experiences as well as those of other lupus patients, it is not at all uncommon for a physician to blame the victim when the diagnosis is unclear.

Though it does not excuse their blaming the patient, I realize that physicians are under a great deal of pressure in trying to make a diagnosis when the potential diagnosis might be lupus. Physicians feel compelled to offer a diagnosis and to treat, but they face several dilemmas. Mistakenly telling the patient that he or she suffers from lupus when symptoms really stem from an inorganic illness or some other organic process would both unnecessarily burden the person with a serious, false diagnosis and mask the true problem. Such a misdiagnosis followed by treatment would expose the patient to the toxic side effects of the drugs used to treat lupus. So a physician wants to be as certain as she or he possibly can be, yet this certainty is the most elusive aspect of lupus.

As I write these words and remember Dr. Smith, my mind flashes forward to more recent events. Dr. Fields. Dr. Gresley. CGH neurology's abandonment of me. I can comprehend some of the reasons why they acted as they did, but I cannot forgive. Not the neurologists at CGH and not Dr. Smith. I cannot release the fury that obliterates insight and destroys peace. But I know the answers do not lie in anger; I will not find the river's source there.

Though I achieved some intellectual insight later, at the time I did not understand, on any level, why Dr. Smith was behaving as she did. All I knew was that I could not find answers or depend on benevolence when dealing with the professionals I had looked to for help and kindness. The summer was drawing to a close. What should I do next? At least I was well insured; I had the financial resources to seek another opinion if I chose to do so. But a part of me began to seriously wonder, "What if Dr. Smith was right, and you're just overanxious? Maybe you're imagining this whole thing."

I had to decide, too, what I was going to do about school. How I had missed my school life during those long, slow days of summer filled with illness, doctors, hospitals, and unanswered questions. But was I strong enough to go back? I could not work a full day in my father's office; I could barely work for a few hours at a time. My endurance for concentrating on my studies was not what it had been. But if I did not return to the university, what would I accomplish by remaining in Maryland? I had found no answers here, no solutions. My hours were empty, and the void had become filled with pain and fatigue. Perhaps if I again filled my time with activities I found meaningful and enjoyable, I could distract my attention from my health problems. This would not make the illness disappear, but at least the sickness would not consume my life. It was time to move forward.

I would have to make a few adjustments. I would only take two classes for the first semester; I would not schedule them for the early morning or in succession. If I built in time throughout the day to rest or go slowly, I thought I could manage. I told my parents that I wanted to return to college, and they agreed.

I did not know then that Mom and Dad had been debating this issue for several weeks. I only discovered recently that Dad was completely against my going back to school. He argued, "How can she function at the university? She can't even work a full day. How can she even think about classes when she's feeling so awful?" But my mom's viewpoint was different. She had sat with me through all the visits to the various doctors. She had seen my life disintegrate into an endless round of tests and physicians. She knew that this was as debilitating as the disease itself. Though, like my father, she was worried and concerned about my health, she strongly felt that I needed to resume a normal life. She convinced my father. Though it was not easy for them, when the fall arrived, my parents did what they thought was best for me. In their love they found the strength to let me go.

Before I left Maryland, my aunt Beth called to tell us about a rheumatologist, a prominent lupus specialist practicing at a large teaching hospital in Philadelphia. A friend of my aunt's had highly recommended this physician. By this time I was less than enthusiastic about visiting yet another doctor, particularly a rheumatologist, but I knew I needed medical help. I made the appointment.

With a sense of freedom and release, I packed my bags for school. But in an uneasy moment, as I was putting clothes in the last suitcase, I wondered what else would be traveling with us in the car loaded with all the possessions that made dorm life complete. What had crept into the folds of my peach comforter, the coils of my toaster, or the rolls of my Monet and Renoir posters? With a toss of my head I shook off the thought, smoothed the soft comforter, and firmly zipped the suitcase closed.

7

Unmasking the Wolf: The Desert Revealed

Fall 1988–Spring 1989

I ARRIVED AT the campus feeling as if I had come home. This was my world. The illness would not invade my life here; I would just not let it. A week after the semester began, my parents once again made the trip to Philadelphia. We celebrated my nineteenth birthday. The next day we went to rheumatologist number three.

When Dr. Kostos entered the examining room where I was waiting for him, I remember thinking that this man looked exactly like Hollywood's stereotype of a doctor. He appeared to be in his early forties and was close to six feet, with a solid but not heavy build. He had thick, wavy gray-and-silver hair and large blue eyes that inspired trust and confidence. He smiled at me, said hello, and gently clasped my hand. Before asking me about my medical history and conducting a physical exam, Dr. Kostos asked me about school and told me that he had a daughter exactly my age who attended Harvard. His pride in his daughter was obvious. As we talked about medical and nonmedical matters, he seemed to be truly listening and interested in what I had to say. After we finished, he asked me to get dressed. He would meet my parents and me in his office.

As my parents and I waited for Dr. Kostos, the tension thickened in the silent room. We all hoped that this time we would find an explanation, a solution. I was so afraid that once again there would be shrugging of shoulders or, worse, blame. As I sat there, I felt a ridiculous urge to flee the hospital. I wondered how far my cash and credit cards could take me. I fantasized about hopping into a cab and heading for the airport and taking a plane—anywhere. Then a vision popped into my head of me running through the airport, trying to keep one of those paper gowns shut while my parents and the doctors chased me, yelling for me to stop. I laughed to myself at the thought and relaxed a bit.

At that moment Dr. Kostos came into the room. After introducing himself to my parents, he took a seat. But he did not choose the doctor's stool, which was at the other end of the room from my parents and me. Instead, he sat down beside me, on the examining table. Taking my hand, his blue eyes looking steadily into mine, he told me that he diagnosed my illness as lupus. He based the diagnosis on my previous lab work, my medical history, and that day's clinical examination. The significant lab results were the positive ANA test and elevated sedimentation rate. When examining me, Dr. Kostos found evidence of arthritis (redness, heat, and swelling in the affected joints); synovitis in my finger joints (inflammation of the connective tissue membrane surrounding the joints); bursitis in the knees (inflammation of the small serous sac between the tendon and bone); a malar rash and a rash on my arms that he believed to be caused by lupus; and oral ulcers. I also had a history of fevers, malaise, and photosensitivity. Dr. Kostos reassured me about the relative mildness of my disease without minimizing my symptoms and the effect they were having on me. In a relaxed, unhurried way, he talked about lupus and answered my and my parents' questions.

Two of the main subjects of concern for us were prognosis and treatment. Dr. Kostos first emphasized that the disease was chronic, not terminal. Then he explained that because lupus could affect any part of the body, there was a long list of problems that *could* occur. Each patient, however, was different, and he could not predict what course any individual's disease would take. As a general, though not at all unbroken, rule, the lupus defined itself within the first year. After that, if the patient had a lupus flare, it would tend to involve the same symptoms and organs. Dr. Kostos recognized the need for treatment in my case, but he did not advocate blasting me with steroids. He wanted to prescribe Plaquenil and start me on a regimen of an NSAID, a nonsteroidal anti-inflammatory drug. He gave me a number of brochures and pamphlets about lupus and introduced me to Ellen Fitzpatrick, a nurse in his office who also conducted the center-city lupus support group meetings. He asked me to schedule an appointment for two weeks hence and told me to call if there were any problems. A trip to the lab and more blood work were required, of course.

Lupus. Latin for "wolf." The name that had inspired such fear and revulsion when I first heard it now brought overwhelming relief. I had a name for this strange collection of symptoms. I no longer felt helpless or out of control. The illness existed. I was not just anxious, crazy, or lazy. I would receive the right treatment, and the symptoms would go away. Now everything would return to normal. "It's over," I thought. Over.

I look back now and wonder how I could possibly have thought that this day marked an end to my health problems. I had much information about lupus stored in my head. I certainly knew that it was a chronic, sometimes deadly disease. But there is a great difference between knowing the facts and making them your own, a part of your reality.

After leaving the hospital, I remember sitting in the car, reading the brochures Ellen had given me. In detail, the pamphlets described the many horrible problems lupus could cause and the sometimes even more dreadful medicines used to treat the disease. But I felt that none of it applied to *me*. It was as if I were reading from a textbook that had been assigned for class. Such a shame for *those* people who suffered in the way described by the text. Yes, I had lupus, but my disease, as Dr. Kostos had said, was "mild." I would never develop all those terrible symptoms. I could not even conceive of it. It seemed as possible as my living on Mars or visiting the moon.

On that day, my parents were also mainly relieved that a diagnosis had finally been made. For them diagnosis held the same meaning as it did for me—power, control. But their relief was mixed with considerable fear. The long list of potential problems became a part of their reality long before it entered into mine. But, in their efforts to protect me, they kept silent about their deepest concerns.

My parents returned to Maryland, and I immersed myself in the familiar, comforting school routine. I did make a few accommodations and changes. My dorm did not have any elevators. I was given a room on the first floor so I would not have to climb the stairs. Washington House is not air-conditioned, so my parents purchased an air conditioner to make the room bearable.

I had received special permission to take only two classes instead of the usual load of four. I regretted not being able to keep up the normal pace. But I had entered Laurel with one year's worth of credits and had planned to graduate in three years. Even if I took only two courses each semester until graduation, I would still complete my degree in four years. In that case, I would be graduating with most of my friends. But I assumed my slowing down was a temporary situation until the medicines took effect. I hoped that I would be able to resume a full-time schedule the next semester, for even though my father could continue to pay for Laurel, my attending the university on a part-time basis for four years would be much more expensive than if I were able to go full time and finish in three. My college education was costly enough, and I did not want to be more of a financial burden on the family.

After receiving the diagnosis, I gathered my circle of friends. These were four girls with whom I had become close the previous year. Teresa was one of them. The other three were Teresa's roommates, Mary, Jessica, and Lily. We had all kept in touch over the summer. We sat in my dorm room, and in a matter-of-fact manner, with a reassuring smile on my face, I explained about the lupus and gave them the brochures the doctor had given me. The news did not come as a shock to them. Over the summer, through phone conversations and letters, I had informed them of my adventures in the medical world, careful to keep my tone light.

But now, with the diagnosis, my disease was more real than it had been when it was nameless. The illness was also easier for my friends to deal with when we were separated by long distances. I look back and see us in that dorm room, five young women, nineteen-year-olds, brought together by friendship. With us, there was a stranger. The lupus. How to deal with its presence? None of us knew. It was something outside our experience. There were awkward pauses. Questions they hesitantly asked such as, "What medicines will you take?" Practical, easy questions that skimmed the surface of all that they were feeling. They wanted to show their support. "If there's anything we can do, you know we're here for you. . . ." But so much was left unsaid on their part and on mine. And that silence, a thing of our own creation, grew over the next months to hurt us all.

The days of that fall semester passed with gathering speed, and my initial euphoria about the diagnosis faded. We began treatment with Plaquenil and an NSAID. Though Plaquenil, a form of quinine, is much safer than steroids, it still carries its own risks, most notably the potential for damage to the retina. Luckily I experienced no side effects from the Plaquenil. But I had a terrible time with the NSAIDs. Their side effects included high blood pressure, severe fluid retention, stomach upset, difficulty breathing, and rashes. Through that fall we tried eight different NSAIDs before deciding to cease and desist.

Even more disturbing than the drugs' side effects was the increasing disease activity. The symptoms with which I had started were more severe.

The arthritis pain worsened, and more joints became involved. When I awoke in the morning and as I moved about during the day, the image of the Tin Man from *The Wizard of Oz* often popped into my head. I felt that I had become the Tin Woman, my limbs painfully stiffened to immobility, my joints rusted by the storms of illness. But I possessed no simple remedy, no can of oil, to restore my limbs to fluid, easy movement.

My stomach problems increased. I lost my appetite and suffered from periodic vomiting, diarrhea, abdominal pain, and almost continual nausea. In the evenings I continued to accompany my friends to the dining hall, because during the week, it was an important social time. We exchanged the news of the day, laughed, debated, and gossiped. Often we were the last group to leave. But many nights I could only manage a bowl of Jello. I was dubbed "The Jello Woman." If I tried anything more adventurous, I paid for it in pain. I would return to my dorm room and lie in bed, writhing until the cramps passed, the medicine took effect, or I threw up. I lost weight all during that semester; it was fortunate that I had some extra pounds to spare.

New symptoms also appeared. I suffered from headaches, including migraines, in which the headache combined with dizziness, nausea, and visual changes. I saw little gray bubbles floating in front of my eyes. There were several other kinds of headaches. The ones I thought of as "the vise" and "the baseball bat" were the worst. Caught in the vise headache, I could almost feel the merciless metal clamped on both sides of my head as some unseen hand squeezed, harder, harder. Or the headache felt as if someone had taken a baseball bat and smashed it against the base of my skull, obliterating everything but my agony.

At no moment of the day and only rarely during the night was I without symptoms. I had night chills and sweats. Frequent bladder infections— nine in a year—including some that were resistant to antibiotics. After every round of the antibiotics, I always developed a yeast infection. Late in the fall, I was diagnosed with Raynaud's phenomenon—a narrowing of the blood vessels in the fingers and toes that causes the extremities to turn white, then blue, and finally red or purple as blood flow returns to normal. Exposure to cold or stress are two common triggers of Raynaud's attacks.

Chest pain and shortness of breath were two more of my symptoms. I spent many nights propped up on pillows, almost sitting upright in my attempts to breathe more comfortably and ease the chest pain. For me there was no more isolating feeling than sitting alone in the middle of the night, watching the clock, as I was borne toward morning on the hands of my pain and the struggle to breathe. I was told that my chest pain and shortness of breath were caused by arthritis in the breastbone.

I suffered from numbness, tingling, tremoring, and weakness in my hands. The doctor ascribed my symptoms to carpal tunnel syndrome and gave me splints to wear at night. I remember going to the main gathering room in our dorm. I sat down at the piano, turning to music, my mother's gift to me. But when I placed my hands on the keys, they felt strange and foreign to my fingertips. I knew the keys were beneath my fingers, but it was as if there were a layer of padding between my fingers and the keys. I tried to play "Summertime," Gershwin's lovely lullaby. But my hands shook too hard for me to hit the keys accurately, and my fingers were too weak to consistently produce sound when I pressed down on the keyboard. My hands no longer stretched far enough to span the keys I needed to form the chords. My fingers tingled as if they had gone to sleep and were just coming awake. I stayed at the piano awhile longer, then left, my music gone from me.

I had been working on a piece of needlepoint, a scene depicting a unicorn standing majestically in a forest. I still remember the colors, the purest white for the unicorn's body and tail and silver for the horn. Hues of blue, green, brown, yellow, and orange for the forest. But unable to pass the needle through the canvas, much less thread the needle with yarn, I put the needlepoint away in the closet. My calligraphy pen, too, was banished to the back of a drawer. It seemed that one by one, all my creative outlets were being taken from me.

In order to give my physician accurate information, I kept a journal of my symptoms and medications. I wrote, "I am always in some pain; sometimes it is severe. I think of it like this. The way I turn a fan on high, medium, and low is the way the lupus switches on pain in my body. But we haven't found the off button. I am forgetting what it feels like to be without pain; my whole body is infested with it." As before, though, the pain was easier to bear than the draining fatigue.

In December, Dr. Kostos decided to try a course of IV pulse steroids. In this treatment, one gram of steroids is administered each day for three days, in my case, in the outpatient procedure unit. The infusion takes two hours. The drug carries with it all the side effects of steroids, plus the risk of a rise in blood pressure during the procedure. My mother accompanied me to the treatments. Unfortunately, I experienced only side effects, not relief, from the pulse steroids. My blood pressure rose, and I had terrible headaches.

   Throughout those autumn months, I was slowly coming to realize that the diagnosis of the lupus did not mean the end of my health problems. There were no simple solutions, no quick fixes. Lupus, in its full identity as a serious, chronic illness, was becoming a part of my reality as I understood it. It was during this time that the shadowy image of the illness as the wolf solidified in my mind.

   Once I lived in a magical fairy field
   With few briars and brambles to block my way.
   Flowers swayed sweetly under a gentle sun;
   My field yielded more pleasures each passing day.

   But as I frolicked in youth through the field
   I sensed an enemy's presence close by.
   Fetid breath surrounded me. Though unseen
   His devilish existence I could not deny.

   Disillusioned, I looked round with opened eyes
   To realize that all was unfamiliar to me.
   For my beautiful field was ringed by deep woods
   Where lurked unknown dangers and mysteries.

   My hidden foe spent months stalking me,
   Attacking in stealth. Yet I still could not name
   This foe who made me a helpless victim
   In this unfair and deadly cat and mouse game.

   Bit by bit, I saw the flashing yellow eyes,
   Teeth I shuddered and quailed to see.
   Then one day my long wait was finally over;
   From the fear of the unknown I was set free.

   My enemy was the wolf of limb lean and long;
   He proved more ferocious with each passing day.
   I could not revel in the flowers of the field.
   My joys in life fell into rot and decay.

   But I could not live that way for long;
   With hope's loving strength, I fought the misery.
   I again took some joy in my fragrant field
   Though it was tainted by the monster that hunted me.

Time has passed; the wolf attacks with sharpened claw,
But I gather all my strength and power
To fight the attacker that brings such vicious pain
Until I can send him away to sulk and glower.

And though I hate the wolf with all of my being
He has brought me a gift even through pain.
For the time I spend away from his company
Is filled with joy so pure such as life never contained!

So I will go on to fight my foe
That without kindness or mercy preys.
For I know I have been granted the strength.
The wolf will surrender to me one day.

In my imagination, my illness became the wolf, a sly, sneaky, vicious, mysterious beast. But I discovered that the notion of the lupus as the wolf was not mine alone. It is a powerful and resonant metaphor that lives in the lupus patient and medical community. In published lupus narratives such as Joanna Permut's *Embracing the Wolf,* the title shows the author invoking the metaphor of the wolf to communicate her illness experience. But I think the most vivid and creative lupus-as-wolf imagery can be found in cyberspace, where patients post Web pages and stories, speak in chat rooms, and visit online support groups.

For me, the most fascinating use of wolf imagery is found in the patients' Web pages. The Missouri Chapter of the Lupus Foundation of America (MCLFA) provides a "Links to Lupus" site that lists personal home pages on lupus. "Living with the Wolf," "Battling the Wolf," "Wolfbitten," and "Wolf Within" testify to ways in which those ill with lupus use wolf imagery as a way of speaking about their lupus experiences.

The Web site I find most poignant is "Wolf in Kids' Clothing," a site created by parents whose children are ill with lupus. This site is linked with the MCLFA Pediatric Lupus Board. The parents of these pediatric lupus patients are using the imagery of the wolf, a legacy in metaphor that their children will receive as they come to understand the meaning of their disease. In all the places on the Internet where patients speak of their illness, I am in the world of the wolf.

Physicians bring the image of the wolf to their own writings about the disease. In the science magazine *Discover,* a resident in internal medicine gives an account of a patient who suffers from lupus. The article is entitled

"The Wolf at the Door." Set dramatically in the center of the article's first page is a vivid painting of a muscled, ferocious wolf who is about to sink his sharp fangs into the throat of a woman asleep in a hospital bed. Above the picture is the caption, "For two months a woman lay unmoving, cast into a strange mute world by a wily predator called lupus."

The name "lupus" in association with the disease now known as systemic lupus erythematosus evolved over centuries, beginning with Hippocrates. He told of a terrible illness that corroded the skin of the face in a pattern that resembled the bite of a ravenous wolf. The disease was viewed with great fear and dread. To this day it is uncertain to which specific disease or diseases Hippocrates was referring. But by mid-nineteenth century, a number of writers decided to name this malady, with its distinctive skin manifestation, lupus. At this time the term "lupus" included several distinct diseases. For these nineteenth-century writers, lupus generally meant *lupus vulgaris,* or cutaneous tuberculosis, as it is currently called.

In the 1840s an important feature of the lupus rash was recognized by Ferdinand von Hebra of Vienna. He noticed that the rash, found mostly on the face, especially on the cheeks and nose, assumed the shape of a butterfly. This rash has since become known as the "butterfly rash."

A few years later, Pierre Cazenave attached the description *erythemateux* "characterized by redness" to the disease. (*Erythematosus* is the Latin equivalent.) By this time, the noncontagious disease was made distinct from other contagious diseases causing similar skin problems. The famous physician Sir William Osler further defined the illness by emphasizing its systemic nature. In fact, in some cases, he found the skin to be not at all affected.

As I learned about the history of the disease and how it is currently perceived by others—patients, health professionals and the public—I came to realize that I had to deal with more than just the physical and even emotional complications of a chronic illness. The metaphors and connotations with which lupus is heavily endowed shadowed and defined my experiences. It was only much later, as I studied the subject and reflected on my own illness, that I more fully understood the impact of the many layers of meaning associated with this disease.

While I journeyed through those months of autumn, I was confronted with certain basic issues that are common to all those who suffer from a chronic illness. My decisions about how I would handle these dilemmas shaped my daily life. My choices were never final. They changed from day to day and over the course of the illness. The issues themselves have been the only constant; they are as chronic as the disease itself.

During my travels I mourned, passing through stages of grief: denial, anger, depression, and acceptance. I felt as if a part of me were dying. It seemed as if I were watching helplessly as I disappeared and a sickly, dependent stranger for whom I had no respect was taking my place, stealing my hopes and dreams. But in the beginning I would not admit my anguish and sense of loss, not to myself or to others. I sank the worst of my grief deep in a lake within me, hiding the lake and the stone weight it hid by keeping my attention firmly fixed upon all that had always given me pleasure at school.

I did not mourn alone; my family and friends grieved, each in their own fashion. For the first year after my diagnosis, my zaide denied the chronic nature of my illness by continually asking me if I had been cured yet. Though my father felt angry about the disease, he could not directly express his fury over the injustice of his child's suffering in this cruel, unfair way. I remember walking into the kitchen one day to find my father fuming over my Visa bill. "Do you realize how much you're spending? You better not spend this much next month!" he shouted.

I was hurt and upset, because he had never questioned my spending habits before. I found out from my mother that the root of my father's anger came from my having so many prescription bills on the statement. He was really angry at my having this disease, which was symbolized by my need for the drugs. The bill also reminded him of the drugs' inability to control my symptoms. Concerns about carrying the financial burden of my illness probably contributed to his emotional reaction. Incapable of expressing the real reasons for his anger, he displaced his feelings onto my spending habits.

As we all struggled to come to terms with the illness, there were many occasions during that first year when we misunderstood and hurt one another. In our grief, we turned to one another for help and understanding. But we were each at different stages of mourning. As we reached out to each other, it was as if there was a wide chasm separating us, preventing communication and comfort.

About a year after the diagnosis, together, we were all able to reach an initial acceptance of the illness, although the acceptance was not final. How could it be? My physical state was never constant. Over the next eight years, my family, my friends, and I came to know the pain of health regained and lost, hopes raised and dashed. Our grief endured again as the waves of disease crested and receded in unpredictable tides.

While struggling to accept my illness, I still had to tend to practical matters. If I had been suffering from an acute injury, I could have laid aside my normal activities until I recovered; it would have been possible and socially acceptable. But faced with a chronic illness, I did not have that luxury. I just had to move forward as best I could.

But how to proceed? I found myself shuttling back and forth between the worlds of health and illness. I had to decide how I wanted to make that transition. In the beginning I created a kind of dual existence; with great dedication I tried to keep the two worlds separate. I wanted the part of my life that involved my usual routine of school, family, and social events pure, untainted by my illness. Receiving my medical care off-campus helped maintain the division between my illness and what I thought of as my real, normal life, where I found meaning and joy.

In a sense this was definitely an advantageous way to cope. I was determined not to let the illness subsume me. But this response inevitably involved some denial of the illness and its effect on me. That line of demarcation I drew so firmly between my life as a patient and my life as a student, family member, and friend, was artificial. Though I wished I could, I did not leave my illness behind during my cab ride from the doctor's office or the hospital to the campus. My illness followed me through the gates of the university. When I would come face to face with my illness at school or other places outside the boundaries I had created, I was caught off guard.

A common, and continually awkward collision of my two existences came in the form of the question, "How are you doing?" In the doctor's office, this question was relatively easy to answer. There the setting was firmly established for me to speak of my illness. The interviews proceeded along given lines, and in my role as patient, I followed my cues. But outside the medical realm, the question became a trap door through which the disease entered my healthy world. And once the disease found its way in, there were no formal guidelines about how to discuss it with others.

In fact, this seemingly innocuous question "How are you doing?" involved all kinds of pitfalls. Quickly, I had to evaluate myself and my inquirer. First, how much did this person genuinely want to know? I learned to give different gradations of answers depending upon how much information I thought the person wanted to hear. I tried to supply an answer that would give the least worry. Second, I had my own needs. For the most part, I kept my answers short, fairly general, using humor whenever possible. I craved normality and I spent a great deal of effort and energy trying to secure it. I did not wish to be constantly reminded of my disease. Like most other young adults, I wanted to fit in with my friends, not to be singled out as different—at least not in this way. But my attempt to pass for normal came at a cost. I was feeling lonely and isolated despite my active social life, because most of the time, I would not, could not, discuss my illness, and all its attendant alien, frightening experiences, with my friends and family.

When I answered "How are you doing?" with "Just fine" or a quirky anecdote when I had just returned from an unpleasant visit at the doctor's office or was in more than usual pain, my response created an inner dissonance. I felt more alone, unable to communicate my illness experiences in any way that I found acceptable. I wanted an answer that would release some of my own worries and concerns without placing a burden upon or inviting the pity of my listener.

In some instances, I found that people avoided asking me "How are you?" by saying "You look so wonderful. You must be feeling better. Generally, they meant well. Implied in these words was the wish for me to feel better. But this greeting invalidated my suffering on the days when I was not feeling better. Sometimes this greeting was a way to forestall me from saying anything about my illness. Mostly, I just said thank you, but this left me feeling empty.

Particularly in the beginning, I made mistakes which caused me regret later. I underestimated or overestimated the amount of detail for which the person was really asking. One professor who lived in my dorm and knew about my medical condition asked me, "How are you doing?" The disease activity had been mounting, and I had been reacting badly to yet another NSAID. I had just come from the doctor's office, and I had not quite readjusted to being back on campus. I supplied her with all the details, and then some, in a monologue probably lasting for a good ten minutes. I realized later that the question had been a polite reflex. She got much more than she bargained for, and she never asked me again.

Eventually, I did resolve this conflict by converting my answers to an inner scale. In my mind, I translated the answer "Fine, thank you" to "I feel lousy but no worse than normal." "O.K." signified "I'm feeling worse than usual." "Not so good" meant that I was probably on my way to the emergency room. Over the months, my parents, my brother, and a few friends came to know my code, which made the question "How are you?" less stressful to answer.

Disclosing my diagnosis and information about the disease to those who did not know of my illness posed another set of complex problems. As a chronically ill person, disclosure was one of the basic dilemmas I faced every day. Whom should I tell? How much? When? In what way should my illness be revealed? These questions were, and are, far from trivial, for disclosure of a chronic illness involves great risks. The ill person might find him or herself shunned or abandoned, particularly if the disease, such as AIDS, carries a strong stigma. As I met others who were chronically ill and also researched the subject, I learned that the ways in which the chronically ill disclose their disease vary widely for any given person, disease, and social situation. The responses also depend on the stage of the illness, both in physical and emotional terms. For example, how someone discloses his or her illness changes as he or she moves through the grief cycle.

I found that the first obstacle to overcome when I told someone about my diagnosis and illness was the general lack of public awareness concerning lupus. Not only did I have to reveal my illness; I also often had to define and explain it. This required extra effort on my part and a delicate gauging of how much information was necessary for the person and the situation.

Though it was aggravating to hear "Lupus? What is it?" when I told someone about my illness, that comment was sometimes more welcome than their responding with, "Oh, yes, lupus. I think I've heard about that." Then a strange, uneasy look would appear in their eyes. I even found that some people moved, involuntarily, I think, a step backward.

I discovered that their reactions resulted from common societal misperceptions about lupus. Lupus is often mistakenly thought of as fatal, a form of cancer, contagious, or related to AIDS. In fact, many pamphlets published by the Lupus Foundation of America address this issue and reassure patients and family members who have heard false information. Nowhere is this more clearly expressed in the "What Is Lupus?" brochure put out by The American Lupus Society (TALS), a west-coast support group that has now merged with the LFA. TALS states emphatically, "Lupus is *not* infectious or contagious. It is *not* a type of cancer or malignancy. Lupus is not related to acquired immunodeficiency syndrome (AIDS)." The "Lupus Fact Sheet" (1998) distributed by the Philadelphia chapter of the LFA gives the information that "Lupus is NOT infectious, rare, or cancerous."

These misperceptions about lupus can seriously affect the ill person's social interactions. The association of lupus with AIDS can stigmatize the ill person. The perception of the disease as terminal can isolate the person ill with lupus. People who do have terminal illnesses often suffer from social isolation as friends who cannot cope distance themselves. The fear of contagion can drive others away from the ill person.

In my own experience, I found out that when Sang and I were undergraduates at Laurel, Sang's mother was upset about his visiting me in Maryland. Though he tried to reassure her that lupus was not contagious, she remained unconvinced and practically forbade him to come. He rarely defied his parents, but he did on this occasion. When I found out what had happened from another mutual friend, I was shocked. I also valued Sang's friendship even more. It was a glimpse of the friend Sang would be to me eight years later when he stayed with me for the weekend at my parents' house in Doylestown.

Because of the public's lack of awareness of or misperceptions about the disease, I had an even greater incentive to conceal my illness. When I did confide my illness to others, I learned to include a comment about its not being contagious. I would smile and say, "Of course, you know it's not catchy." We would laugh as if it had not even been an issue, but I often saw relief in the other person's expression. I know my addressing the other person's concern in this casual way was an important part of my revealing my diagnosis. I would also stress that this was a chronic, not a fatal, disease, and that there were treatments if not cures. My tone was always optimistic. I attempted to disclose my illness to others in such a way so that I conveyed the necessary information while calming people as much as possible and not frightening them away.

The way I coped with disclosure altered over the years. In the beginning, when I was still coming to terms with the lupus, I mostly kept silent, at times going to great lengths to keep my illness hidden. I did not like to acknowledge its existence. I feared the reactions of the person I told. I did not wish to drive people away, but neither did I want their pity. I wanted people to see me as I wished to see myself—strong, independent, and whole. Not speaking of the lupus or allowing it to become a part of new relationships was an attempt to maintain control over my life, another setting of boundaries.

I also did not often disclose my illness because I was worried that I would not be believed. At that time, like many lupus patients, I was invisibly chronically ill. In fact, the butterfly rash and the continual fevers lent me a deceiving glow of good health. I received continual compliments on my rosy cheeks and beautiful complexion. When I did try to explain that my heightened color was the result of illness and that I suffered from chronic health problems, I was often met with frank disbelief. "But you look so healthy!" was the frequent response.

But in some ways, this cloak of invisibility was quite beneficial, because I avoided the labels of illness or disability and the stigma and social isolation that often result. I was spared the embarrassing questions the noticeably ill or disabled receive. I believe that my being invisibly chronically ill permitted me to move more easily between the worlds of health and illness. I think that the invisibility of my illness drew me more, on an emotional level, into the world of the healthy. Do we not see ourselves, at least partially, through others' eyes? When others perceived me as normal, it was easier for me to do the same and carry on in the everyday world defined by health. It helped me to fight against becoming trapped in the world of illness.

Though for the most part I chose to keep quiet about the lupus, the accommodations that I needed for me to remain in school forced me to reveal my illness to the people who had the power to make those accommodations. As I have already mentioned, my dorm room had to be on the first floor, and I could take only two classes a semester instead of the usual four. To fulfill those needs, I had to tell the housemaster and the dean about my illness. I also had to talk about my illness with my professors if I needed an extension. Sometimes, because the arthritis in my fingers prevented me from writing at a normal speed, I asked for more time to take an exam.

Frequently these arrangements invited questions from other students. In my dorm, some students asked why I had been put at the top of the lottery and been given the single on the first floor. When I would meet a new student, and we would ask one another about our course schedule, I had to decide how I would explain my taking only two courses. Students in my class sometimes wanted to know why I had been given extra time to complete a paper or take an exam. There were many other similar situations in which the person posed a question which gave me the choices of confiding about my illness, giving a vague answer, or lying.

I found it most difficult of all to confide my secret to my professors and to the men I was dating—probably because both kinds of relationships involved my identity and self-conception, though in very different ways. I prided myself on doing my best to fulfill my responsibilities at school without any special favors, but sometimes I did need extensions on papers or makeup exams. In that case I had to inform my professor of my condition. I detested doing that. In the classroom I was learning the material, but I was also becoming initiated into the academic world where I hoped someday to be a professional. I needed to be seen as a potential member of that group. I worried that I would be looked upon differently because of my lupus, that my professors would not believe in my future as a scholar in quite the same way. I wanted to be judged on the quality of my work, not on my disease.

I was also concerned that the professor might think I was taking advantage of the situation, or even making the whole thing up. There is always an astounding outbreak of both exotic and more mundane sicknesses around exam time. My healthy appearance complicated the situation further. By junior year I had resolved this problem by talking to the professor at the beginning of the semester. In a very casual way, I would say, "I wanted to let you know about some chronic health problems of mine. I have lupus. Have you ever heard of it?" I would give a little information about the disease if the answer was no, then continue, "This probably won't come up again all semester, but just in case, I didn't want it to come out of left field." For the most part, my professors were extremely appreciative of my coming to them in this way. At least they knew that if I did ask for extra time or an incomplete, I was being honest. Also, I did not approach my professors until a few weeks into the semester. I mentioned my illness only to those professors I felt would be receptive. As for the others, I hoped that it would not become necessary to explain missed classes or request extensions.

It was always difficult to tell a man I was dating about the illness. During the first year, I lied. One date asked me how I had spent the previous summer. Too ashamed to admit that I had not really been working, studying, or spending my time in an otherwise productive fashion, I told one date that I had worked in my father's software company. On another occasion, I was walking with him through the center of campus, up a brick path known as Laurel Walk. My arthritis was bothering me, and I was tired. But instead of explaining, I invented an errand in the opposite direction. As soon as he was out of sight, I limped into a building to rest. Though I also often kept my illness secret in new platonic friendships, as the friendship deepened I would confide in the other person. I rarely lied to my new friend; I just would be vague or evasive in my answers. But I responded differently in my romantic relationships.

Perhaps my memories of Carlos encouraged me to hide my illness from men. He had been my first love. I thought he had genuinely cared for me. If he would not stay, why would someone else, who did not even have a shared history with me when I was healthy? I also think that my not being open with men about my illness involved my efforts to keep alive my self-conception as a whole, sensual woman who could be attractive to men. Again, I was defining borders, drawing boundaries. I was attempting to keep the lupus from infiltrating that part of my life.

Throughout the fall and spring following my diagnosis, I made an enormous effort to cover up my illness and try to pass for a healthy young adult. But I could not keep the illness hidden all the time, and the attempt drained a great deal of precious energy. I do remember one night during the spring semester of that sophomore year. It had been a good day for me. The pain had abated for the moment, and I had some energy. I know that my date, Tom, and I, ate dinner first, but I recall little of that. What does abide is the memory of our wandering through the park by the Delaware River that spring evening. Hands entwined, we stood by the water, which twinkled with the lights of passing boats. His lips touched mine, and in that perfect evening, the illness receded into the darkness, somewhere beyond the river.

A few weeks later, he left for Virginia to begin training in physical therapy. The evening was a gift that reinforced my shaky identity as a woman who could still be attractive to a man and give and take pleasure with her body. But if he had stayed, and we had continued to see one another, I would have needed to tell him of my illness at some point. But when? How? Would he have been angry with me for not saying anything at the beginning? I still had no answers for how I should tell a man with whom I was romantically involved that I had lupus.

Talking about the disease with people who knew and informing those who did not were two constant dilemmas I have continued to face, though they have become easier over time. But an equally troublesome problem was asking for help. For the chronically ill in today's American society, asking for help is a difficult task. Our society places an enormous value on personal independence and autonomy. The role of the family as caretaker for the ill person is not as firmly rooted in our society, which has much weaker kinship ties, as it is in other, less individualistic societies.

The burden of asking for help was made heavier by the values instilled in me by my parents. I had been raised to hold self-sufficiency in high esteem. In my household, to give was always better than to receive. I was worried about becoming a dependent, needy person who would take continually from those around her and not be able to offer anything in return. Would I be able to become the kind of person I and my parents expected me to be? Would I be nothing more than a burden, a disappointment to myself and to others?

Last of all, I grappled with the inherent difficulties of such an unpredictable disease. My condition varied from hour to hour, day to day, month to month, making it harder for me to adjust. When I had even a few good days in a row, my hopes would begin to rise, and I would think of remission. Then I would feel worse, and those hopes would be crushed. I felt as if I were trapped on a wild seesaw; I was helplessly fixed on one end, the disease on the other. The illness was in complete control, and all I could do was try to hold on. My family and close friends rode the seesaw with me, equally powerless to stop the mad ride.

In several ways, the changeability of my disease also made it very problematic to manage the tasks of everyday life. Some days I could do much more than others. My strength and endurance even varied dramatically with the time of day. This made making plans frustrating. I would begin the day with a list of things to do. Sometimes I would be able to complete my list, but other days I would find it impossible to do anything at all. I learned that I had to allow myself much more time to finish what I needed to do. When I was writing a paper or preparing for an exam, I needed to start well ahead of time, because I never knew when I would lose hours or days to the disease. I could not count on my body to function at the last minute.

Nor could I rely on my body to get me to social functions. I always felt guilty making plans with people, because I knew that there was a real possibility I would have to cancel. But I was not going to say no when I was invited to go places. I was determined not to be a hermit.

The variations in disease activity also meant that my family, my friends, and I could not settle into any routine of giving and asking for help. Often friction occurred after a period in which my symptoms had been more severe. People, usually my parents, wanted to continue giving me the same amount of assistance even though it was no longer necessary. But I did not want to be coddled. At other times I had difficulty getting the help I needed because I was not believed. Someone might say, "Well, you look fine. Besides, I saw you walking around campus this morning, and you seemed all right then. How can you be so sick now?"

Especially during that first year after my diagnosis, as I explored the unfamiliar territory of chronic illness, facing all these issues along the way, I found lupus support group meetings to be quite useful. The group shared practical information about the disease and treatments. Most of the time I found solace in the meetings. I was no longer alone, feeling like a freak of nature. Here was a place where, for a few hours, I did not have to conceal the presence of the illness. In that atmosphere of freedom and openness, I could share my illness experiences and voice my concerns and frustrations. We could offer each other comfort born of our common knowledge of what it was like to suffer with the disease—a knowledge that none of our family and friends, no matter how much they cared for us, could really possess.

But as much as I did value the meetings, I felt that there was a gap between me and most of the members of the group. Yes, we all suffered from lupus, but I was much younger than the majority of the group. Most of the members tended to be women in their early thirties to mid-forties. For the most part, they were married, had children, and were trying to balance their illness, families, and jobs. I had just turned nineteen. I was at a very different point in my life. I was worried about finishing school, beginning my career, and eventually marrying and having children. I wanted to find other young people in a similar position. So I decided to put an ad in my school newspaper and start a lupus support group of my own.

I got responses to my ad, but the other students were usually ambivalent about getting too involved with any kind of regular meetings. We often spent a long time on the phone. Once in a while, another student with lupus and I would meet a few times, just the two of us. Our relationships with our parents were a frequent topic of conversation. Some students felt that their parents were overprotective; others felt that their parents were not understanding enough about the limitations the disease imposed. What most clearly united us, though, were our efforts to keep up, both socially and academically. The other students seemed to be experiencing the same intense pressure I did to maintain a healthy, normal college lifestyle. Regular lupus support group meetings would intrude upon that lifestyle. But at the same time, they wanted to talk, at least occasionally, with another young adult who knew the pain of living with a chronic illness.

There was one notable exception to this general hesitancy to become a part of a lupus support group. A graduate student, Cheryl. Her call marked the beginning of a close friendship that lasted until she moved away from the city six years later. She and I attended the regular support group meetings together and commiserated when we arrived home after a doctor's appointment. Had we been healthy and our paths had crossed, I do believe we would have become friends. We shared similar interests, and our conversations ranged over subjects well beyond our medical condition. But there was an added depth of communication between us, for we knew that when we did discuss the lupus, we would be understood.

We have lost touch now, but I still think of her, most often in my dreams. When we meet there, I know without asking that the lupus is gone from her. She is well. She is slim and svelte, no longer bloated and swollen from steroids. Moving with agile grace, she comes to sit beside me and tells me of all that has happened in her life since we have last spoken. Sometimes her face looks so much like my own. I know that I am dreaming for us both, wishing for the day when the lupus is no more.

As I traversed the alien land of chronic illness, the people close to me were doing the same. I was extremely lucky. The circles formed by my friends and family remained unbroken. For my part, I chose not to withdraw from the people in my life. Some chronically ill people do, from shame or embarrassment, isolate themselves from others. For their part, my friends and family stayed by my side. But in many cases of chronic illness, friends do drift away. Sometimes it is because the ill person cannot keep up with the activities in which he or she used to be involved. Serious illness can be particularly difficult for friends of ill young adults, for ongoing disease is usually not a part of a young adult's experiences. The young also believe, on some level, that they will live forever, in strength and health. Faced with the fear of the unfamiliar and a challenge to their assumptions, young adults can abandon their ill friend.

My family's and my friends' loyalty and caring did not mean, of course, that we all immediately came to some kind of harmonious peace, understanding, or agreement about how we were going to handle the illness. That first year after I was diagnosed was marked by many miscommunications, by screaming and weeping, and by bewildering silences.

My relationship with my parents became strained. Though I had been ill for several months at home, my parents had to adjust to the definitive diagnosis from a distance. While they were attempting to face the illness in their own way, namely, in trying to find ways to keep me safe and give me back my health, I was focused on keeping my life at school intact. In my efforts to protect them as well as maintain a sense of normalcy for myself,

I didn't always tell them about my symptoms or my treatments. When I did inform them, I gave them an abridged, minimized account. My parents sensed or found out about what I was doing, and their imaginations began to riot with horrible images of what I was not saying. In my silences, grew their fears. As they became more frightened, they became more protective. In turn, I felt that they were threatening my cherished independence. I was determined not to become an invalid, dependent child. So the tensions mounted.

My aunt Beth and my brother often acted as effective intermediaries between my parents and me. They listened compassionately and empathetically and presented my parents' point of view in a way that I could understand. Though my parents and I did not come to any real peace until the following summer, my aunt and my brother played an essential role in allowing my parents and me to continue communicating even when the baying of the wolf made it difficult for us to hear each other.

Though by the time we were in high school we had become close, the arrival of the lupus deepened my relationship with my brother. He could have resented the overwhelming amount of attention I was receiving. When one sibling is chronically ill, jealousy and rivalry on the part of the healthy sibling can be the result. But Jonathan responded only with unreserved, unconditional love. He supported me with encouraging words and concrete acts. Engraved in my memory is the image of my brother walking beside me, his long, strong legs effortlessly matching their stride to my slow, unsteady gait, while others rushed ahead of us.

My friends coped with my illness in various ways. Rachel, the friend who a few years later accompanied me to the Broadway show in December, immediately went to the library to research lupus. She said later that she did not want to bother me with all kinds of questions that I might not want to answer, but that she needed to gather information about the disease for both our sakes. She felt that she could not help me as a friend without knowledge of the disease. She was also seeking relief for her own fears. The unknown, no matter how terrible, is more terrifying than the known. It certainly did not reassure her when her mother, upon hearing the news that I had lupus, asked, "Is Melissa going to die?"

Rachel was attending a college in upstate New York at the time, but our phone calls were frequent. She showed her concern and support and spoke freely of the illness, encouraging me to do the same, though she was always careful not to dwell on it. Two other childhood friends were also early confidants. Jennifer attended college in Baltimore. She was a gifted and faithful letter writer, and we corresponded often. Minh and I also wrote to each other. Both Minh and Jennifer lacked any inhibitions when it came to talking about lupus.

Such was not the case with my friends at school. Throughout that fall and spring semester following the diagnosis, they maintained a general, blanketing silence about the lupus. If I did try to mention it, they changed the subject. I began to think of the lupus as the "L-word." I knew I could let off a string of four-letter expletives, and no one would bat an eyelash, but God forbid I should let the word "lupus" out of my mouth. One evening at dinner, early in the fall of 1988, we were in the dining hall, and an acquaintance who was not a member of our immediate circle came to sit with us. He did not know about my illness. He offered me some food I was not permitted to eat. When he asked me why I could not have it, a friend quickly jumped in. "She has an allergy," she interjected, then engaged him in conversation. I was fuming. I probably would not have said anything, but would it have been so terrible if I had mentioned lupus? Was it that much of a disgrace? I felt that it should have been my choice to tell or not to tell.

As I recall this time in my life, I come across another snapshot memory. I am in my college room, my first home away from the house in which I had grown up. This small space has always given me peace and pleasure, for it is the first place that I, as a young woman, have made my own. Now, as I gaze through the window, I see and hear Mary and a group of our friends on their way to the Saturday football game. They are laughing in the bright sunlight of the Indian summer day. I was not invited. Why? Are my friends embarrassed by me? How could they not be? I am ashamed of myself. This answer comes from some part of me I did not even know was there. Sitting there in the room, I feel as if I am trapped in a dim prison. I press my fingers to the glass, a seemingly impenetrable barrier between me and my friends and the life I had before the lupus.

A turning point came in November. It was a Saturday night, and a number of us were gathered in someone's dorm room watching a movie. I began to experience severe, cramping abdominal pain and nausea. I also felt feverish. Jessica asked a few times, "Melissa, are you all right?" I repeatedly told her that I was just fine. Determined not to allow the symptoms to end my evening early, I stayed until the last credits flickered off the screen. Finally I went back to my own room, though I never went to sleep that night. By morning I knew I had to go to the emergency room. As luck would have it, a fierce rainstorm was flooding the campus. I would not have been able to get to the cab without becoming completely drenched. I was always losing my umbrellas and was currently without one. So I called the girls (Jessica, Mary, Teresa, and Lily) to ask if they could lend me an umbrella.

Jessica told me that I could borrow her umbrella and that she would bring it down to my room. After she handed me the umbrella, she asked, "Where are you going in this downpour?" I confessed my destination. She was already supposed to be on her way somewhere else and was therefore unable to go to the emergency room with me, so she called back upstairs and arranged for Teresa to accompany me to the ER. With my permission, after I left, she telephoned my mom. Later, my mother informed me that Jessica had been quite distressed. She told my mom, "My God, why couldn't she have told us she was that sick? I saw something was wrong last night, and I kept asking her if she was O.K. She said she was fine, but I knew she wasn't. We're her friends. Doesn't she know that?" Teresa sat in the emergency room for several hours until my bladder infection was diagnosed and treatment was begun. It was the first bladder infection I had ever experienced, so I did not recognize the symptoms. When I returned home, my other friends called or visited to check on me and see if I needed anything. During that episode I realized my friends were not drawing away from me. They did care. Their silence about the lupus was filled with meaning and emotion, but their actions and their inability to discuss my illness did not signify embarrassment or a wish to be rid of me.

It was not until the end of the summer that we really came to more fully understand each other and completely break the silence. But gradually, through the rest of the fall semester and the following summer term, during the school year we achieved small insights and were able to communicate our feelings and needs better. Mary seemed to be having the most difficulty dealing with my illness. She refused to talk about it, and it was she who most often would not include me in certain activities. I can remember her seriously asking me how I was feeling only once, in the fall at a party, before I made my visit to the emergency room. Mary had already downed several glasses of the Jamaican rum Teresa had brought from her home in Kingston. Mary was well on her way to being drunk, and I thought, "Why can't she ask me this question and cope with my answer when she's sober?"

Later, a few weeks after I had gone to the emergency room, Jessica told me that a girl in Mary's high school had died of lupus. I realized that Mary's behavior stemmed from fear. Though I had said that lupus was not fatal, her early and only other experience with lupus indicated otherwise. I decided that I needed to speak with her. But when the moment came, I could not bring myself to address her deepest worries. Could it have been because, at some level, I shared them? I could have offered her some reassurance. Medically defined, my lupus was mild, because it did not involve any major organs, but I could not offer any guarantees that this would not change.

So I did not speak to her about the girl she knew in high school. I contributed my own unspoken words to the general silence. But I did question Mary about why she did not invite me to football games and various other social events. She explained that she did not want me sitting in the football stadium underneath the hot sun for several hours. She did not ask me to other events if she thought they might be too tiring for me. I told Mary, and the other girls so that Mary would not feel singled out, that it was imperative for me to do as much as possible within the limits of the illness. Most important, I needed to be the one to decide what I could and could not do. I appreciated their concern, but I did not want them to make decisions for me.

The visit to the emergency room may have brought about a better understanding between me and my friends, but that stormy November Sunday marked an escalation in the tensions between me and my parents. When my parents found out the way that I handled, or mishandled, getting treatment for the infection, they exploded. First, they were angry that I had delayed going to the hospital. People ill with lupus are more susceptible to infection. Infection can also trigger the lupus. Therefore, infections must be treated quickly. I was lucky that the problem was not a serious one that would have required more immediate attention. My parents were furious that I had not confided in anyone. It was difficult enough for them to be so far away and not to be able to take care of me. I was making it worse by not asking for help when I needed it from those around me. They thought of me as being alone, and it terrified them.

Why did I refuse to end the evening early that Saturday even though by then I was nauseous, running a high fever, and in a great deal of pain? Why did I not seek treatment earlier? Part of the answer lies in my not fully accepting my disease at this point. If I did not acknowledge my symptoms, then they were not real. By staying through the movie, I was drawing my boundaries again, keeping the disease out of my social time. Why did I not admit that I needed help? Perhaps my asking for the umbrella was a roundabout way of doing just that. After all, if I had been that determined to do without assistance, I could have just gotten soaked. But asking for help was an overwhelming obstacle for me then, and even now, though to a lesser extent. It seemed a sign of weakness and made me ashamed and embarrassed. I was also protecting my friends, keeping them from worry. And though I did not openly acknowledge it, even to myself, a tiny part of me, buried deep, felt that I must maintain a healthy facade, or I would lose my friends. No single explanation or emotion lay behind my behavior. Sociology texts make the grieving process sound so organized—a clear, coherent, step-by-step map that one follows. But human experience is rarely that easily categorized.

I apologized to my parents and promised that I would not wait to be treated the next time and would also ask for help. I did learn from my mistakes, not repeating them as often. But my promise did not completely resolve the situation. I still was not acknowledging my illness. I was also intensely involved with keeping up at school, both socially and academically. None of this changed after my trip to the emergency room. I was not ready to alter my behavior completely. My parents were now even less confident in my ability to manage my own illness. They became more protective. They constantly called to probe and question; I could hear the worry in their voices. They believed that school was too much activity, too much pressure. In turn, I felt that my independence was increasingly at risk.

My relationship with my parents reached a crisis with the arrival of the Christmas holidays. My parents wanted me to take a leave of absence for the next semester. They said that they did not want me to give up school permanently. They just thought that I would benefit from some rest. I adamantly refused to go back to Maryland. I felt that since lupus was chronic, rest would not make my disease disappear. I needed to learn how to live with my disease, not retreat by going to my parents.

These were the arguments we used, but there were other emotions and issues underlying our debates. I needed the continuity of Laurel. My world was falling apart, and my last bastion of normalcy was my role as a student. I clung tenaciously to college like a life raft. Also, school meant moving ahead, into my future. My parents were and would always be an important part of my life, but not in the same way as they had been while I was growing up. Their house was a place to be visited on vacations; it was no longer my home. Returning to Maryland meant stagnation, even regression. Though I was an ill young woman, I was still a young adult, not a child. And I remembered only too well those awful months before I was diagnosed.

To my parents, school was where I was alone and vulnerable, assaulted by the fatigue and stress of my studies and my social life. I would be well, in what they defined as my home, in Maryland, where they could keep me safe and protected as they had when I was a child.

We fought. My mother and I cried and pleaded with each other. My dad yelled. My aunt, brother, and even grandparents mediated. This was a wrenching time for both my parents and me. We had always enjoyed a peaceful and uncomplicated relationship. My teenage years were uneventful. My parents granted me a great deal of freedom, and I did not abuse it. Our relationship had been founded on trust, love, and shared values and understandings. When we did disagree, we resolved our differences quickly. Serious conflict was not a part of our relationship. But I felt the need to stay in school too deeply to acquiesce to their demands, as much as I hated to argue with them. Finally, my dad threatened that he would not pay my tuition. I could not have paid for school. At that point my rheumatologist intervened, recommending that my parents allow me to stay in school. He told them that while a rest certainly would not hurt me, leaving school for the semester could harm me psychologically. My parents took his advice. I won my battle and was able to remain in school.

Several years later, my mother and I spoke of this time in our lives. She admitted to me that her fury, worry, and heartbreak were mixed with respect for the strong, independent young woman I had become. She knew what it had taken for me to defy her and my father. And it was with a bittersweet joy and pride that she recognized her child grown.

Looking back now, I understand the significance of that December, for both my parents and me. I crossed over the threshold from childhood into adulthood. Lupus defined the moment for me and my parents. But the time would have come had I not fallen ill. I have watched my friends, who enjoy perfect health, make the same transition. The issues that marked their passage from one stage of life to another were different for each of them. But, as it must, the moment of separation came to them all.

I returned to school for the spring semester, feeling the heavy weight of my parents' accusations and fears that I should not be going back. During the semester all my usual symptoms became more severe. I ran constant fevers, averaging about 100°, but often rising to 102°. The fatigue was sometimes overwhelming. The arthritis became more painful, particularly in my hips, and I developed tendinitis in my shoulders. Sores appeared on my scalp. Of particular concern to me and my physician, were my stomach problems.

But I managed to finish the spring term. My family, my friends, and I had passed those first nine months after the diagnosis attempting to accept my illness and integrate it into our lives. This involved far more than our efforts to construct a daily routine or communicate with one another. For me and those who shared my life most intimately, the illness evoked powerful questions of meaning. Why is there suffering? Why are we mortal? Why is there injustice? Is there any fairness in the universe—some system of checks and balances? We all responded to these questions in various ways, attempting to find order in chaos and significance in senselessness. I also wondered how the illness would change me and the way I conceived of myself. With the wolf traveling with me, who would I be, where would I go, and how would I get there?

8

Journeying East

Fall 1988–Summer 1989

I FOUND solace and answers in my writing, especially my poetry. Poetry served me in my illness in the same way that it always had—as a means of understanding my experiences and reaching out to others. When the disease entered my life, I became trapped in a muddy whirlpool of emotions and questions. Caught up in an issue, event, emotion, or problem, images would come to me. As I achieved greater insight, the images would become sharper, gaining clarity much like a photograph in a developing solution. From these pictures, using both my intellect and my emotions, I created my poems.

Comparing my past to my present was one issue that preoccupied me during those early months. I looked back to what I used to be able to do and could not anymore. One thing I missed was dancing. I never was a fantastic dancer, but I had been passable, perhaps on occasion even graceful. How I loved to dance and feel the music, whether it was sweet and slow, or quick and pulsating, flow through me as I moved about the floor! Now my movements felt jerky and uncoordinated. I was in too much pain and too tired to dance.

> I love the night.
> For in my dreams, healthy and whole
> I dance with light and painless steps,
> or race down a hill in summer,
> moving with effortless, graceful ease.
> How hard it is to come awake,

descend with a thump
into a stiff, awkward body.
Though I cannot run, except in dreams,
I still welcome the day, call it friend
for all the joys and pleasures
it brings to me even in the midst of pain.
Life needs both day and night to be complete.
Though I wish that one night I could bring strength
and health back with me from the realm of sleep
to keep with me through all the hours of the day.
Then I would not have to wait for a dream to dance.

Later in that first year, I came to a deeper acceptance of the need to give up the past and live in the present moment, learning to embrace the pleasures of the day instead of dreaming of what was gone.

I stood at the gate helplessly looking in,
Yearning to be once more in my field.
The gate mocked me with its toothless grin,
Saying, "You may look, but I will never yield."

For this field was my treasured past
Filled with beauty, joy, and delight.
How soon it all escaped my grasp—
This field that was so sparkling and bright.

I used to rollick by that stream—over there,
By trees that offered their fruit to the sky.
The flowers of my field were beyond compare;
Very few times did the sun say good-bye.

Reluctantly I turned my eyes
From that vision that tormented me
To look at what I couldn't deny:
Future's landscape blighted by disease.

Verdant green once carpeted this land;
Fragrant blooms formed a tapestry.
God gave beauty with a generous hand.
All was gone so suddenly.

For now all the blossoms were dead,
Withered corpses of hopes and dreams.
Black colored the landscape instead.
How dreary and arid this place seemed!

In agony I fell to the ground,
Both landscapes searing my soul with pain.
But at that moment, as I looked down,
Wonder bathed me in a soothing rain.

A flower rose before me,
So radiantly golden of hue
The desert ahead, the field behind
Blessedly receded from my view.

I this flower's acquaintance made,
Learning more as each day passed by.
Soon she let me know her name—
Laughter—I tried to keep her by my side.

Soon another flower came into sight;
This one was different it is true.
But she had beauty in her own right.
Friendship is the name she used.

In astonishment I could suddenly see
That in my misery, I had been blind.
I had a whole garden surrounding me,
The Present, a place where peace I could find.

As I explored my garden each day,
At last I found the very best blooms.
They help to keep grief at bay;
Hope and Love are best at driving away gloom.

So I find myself keeping my garden;
Sometimes it is hard to tend.
But I now know that it has always been
The only garden that is ours in the end.

The need to live in and value the present moment is a guiding principle
I still live by. But it was not as if I experienced an epiphany that brought a

simple and final acceptance of my illness. As the disease progressed, my garden of present moments was sometimes completely, even hideously, transformed. In this new place I was often tempted to look backward to the past and forward to the future, mourning both. Eventually, though, I would use my gardening tools of laughter, friendship, hope, and love to till the soil and create a new present garden in which I could find happiness.

Though I had been given an acute awareness of the uncertainty of the moment and the need to take the days as they came, I was, as a young adult, at a very future-oriented part of my life. I was in school, preparing with great excitement for my career. In the next ten years I hoped to marry and start a family. Lucky for me, I often thought, the career of writer, researcher, and academic did not require any special physical prowess. I felt blessed that my chosen profession was still within my reach. The belief that I would continue on my life path sustained me.

Since I did not know what the lupus held in store for me, and the doctors could not make any reliable predictions, I planned for my future as best I could, following the route I had set for myself, telling myself that I would deal with any slow spots or detours as they came. Meanwhile, I tried to live most fully in my present moments. I was really living only as we all do, as vulnerable human beings whose futures are not under our full control. The knowledge of the precariousness inherent in life comes to us all, each in our own time. I was just confronted with this knowledge earlier than I might otherwise have been.

My poetry was a way for me to deal with my illness by gaining insights about what was happening to me, but my poems were also a way to share my illness experiences. When the poem left my hands and was given to another, I often formed a link to that other person, a bond formed out of understanding. I was brought out of the isolation into which chronic illness often thrusts the sick person and which can be worse than any physical pain. I offered my poems to a few friends and family. Sometimes the poems opened dialogue between us. My poetry created a pathway of communication by which we could tell each other of our pain instead of hiding our feelings behind forced jocularity, displaced anger, or silence.

I also gave a few poems to my rheumatologist. He was the first physician with whom I shared my poetry. I wrote in my journal, "I just wrote some poetry today about the lupus; I used the metaphor of the wolf. . . . Maybe I'll show it to the doctor. My poetry has always been such a basic part of who I am. What better way for him to know and understand me? And he must know me to help me. For he is treating me—not the disease."

Later I discovered, much to my surprise, that he had given the poems to his nurse, Ellen Fitzpatrick. She told me that he had been very impressed by them. Ellen in turn passed them around to others. When I met her with a nursing student in the hall one day, after Ellen had introduced me, the student exclaimed, "Oh, you're the one who wrote 'The Wolf' and 'The Garden'! I really enjoyed those poems."

Through the exchange of poetry, my doctor and I were building the kind of open relationship in which I felt more comfortable reporting my symptoms. My experiences in the pre-diagnosis phase, especially with Dr. Smith, had made me wary about confiding too much. But it was essential to be honest when I told my physician about my symptoms. Though there are blood tests that are used to indicate lupus activity, they are not definitive. My rheumatologist relied mainly on my reported history and the clinical exam to decide how we should treat.

In these ways, poetry became a vital part of my illness experience. Poetry is built out of metaphor. I used the power of metaphor to connect myself with others and create a torch to illuminate my world so that I might find beauty and meaning in it. Through metaphor I negated my illness, rejecting the loneliness and chaos that chronic illness brings.

Susan Sontag, the author of the now classic essay "Illness as Metaphor," vehemently argues that the act of making illness metaphors can and should be stopped. She states that throughout history, we have associated certain metaphors with particular illnesses, and that this practice places undue hardship and suffering on ill people.

Some illness metaphors are harmful. But, as I have seen from my own experience, they can also bring comfort, connection, and understanding—for patients, their loved ones, and health-care practitioners. For what is the making of metaphors but an attempt to understand one thing by relating it to another that is known and familiar? This is one of our most basic thought processes. To me, the association of metaphors with serious illness seems entirely natural. Illness causes us to ask fundamental questions of meaning in which we try to make the incomprehensible comprehensible. Faced with the suffering of illness, we turn toward metaphor for explanation and solace.

Across time and cultures, people have created illness metaphors to make sense of their experiences. The specific meanings and metaphors are diverse, but the process of questioning and assigning metaphors to disease remains the same. Illness metaphors are too deeply rooted for us to exterminate them. And we should not try. Like any tool, illness metaphors can be used to create or to destroy. One can use a hammer to help build a home in which to live; one can also use a hammer to kill. It is for us to decide.

Though my writing became an essential way for me to understand and cope with my illness experiences, I still felt a basic lack. It was not something that I dwelt upon, but I wanted . . . something. . . . I remember roaming about the city on a weekday afternoon. I was troubled about my illness and was hoping to find peace and forgetfulness in my walk. I came upon a small Catholic church tucked into a corner of a block. In the stillness and quiet, I stood at the black wrought-iron gate that surrounded the church and its cheerful, colorful garden which a priest was tending. As he turned to go back into the church, he saw me and gave me a quizzical smile. I yearned to follow him into the church, to fill the emptiness I felt so acutely at that moment. But I only returned the smile and went on my way.

Religion had never played a significant role in my life. My parents had sent me to Hebrew school and even made sure that when I turned thirteen I had a Bat Mitzvah, a rite of passage for Reform and Conservative Jewish females that marks the passage from childhood to adulthood. But the spiritual meaning of our religion was never really discussed or emphasized at home. My parents provided me with access to Judaism, but the decision of if, or how, I would incorporate it into my own life, was left up to me. My parents gave me a clear moral, ethical code to live by, but it did not come from Judaism. In fact, as I grew older, my father did not hide his hatred of all organized religions, including his own. My mother was a spiritual person who believed in God, but her faith encompassed and reached beyond the tenets and beliefs of Judaism. As for me, I often tried to sense the presence of God in the synagogue, hear His voice as the cantor chanted the ancient words from the Torah, but I never heard or felt anything.

Growing up, I had a friend, Kim, who was a devout Christian. Her religion gave her life shape. Her faith was a thing of beauty. It did not make her smug or judgmental. Instead it radiated from her and endowed her with a profound serenity and sureness that I did not possess. When her grandmother died, Kim mourned, but her beliefs sustained her. I wondered what I would hold onto if I suffered some awful loss. I had been taught not to have faith but to question the basic nature of the world around me. Most of the time, I was grateful for the freedom of mind and heart that my parents had bestowed upon me. I could be open to ideas, feelings, and experiences my friend could never know. And I often thought, "What if she's wrong?

How can she be that certain?" The answer was faith, but I did not comprehend that then, not with my soul. Nor did I understand it years later as I walked the streets of Philadelphia, feeling an ache, a void for something I could not even name.

As I attempted to find meaning in my experiences, so did my family and closest friends. When I became ill, my mother became furious with God. She shouted up to him that she would not pray to Him or enter a synagogue until I was healed. Why should He have visited this sickness upon me?

My father did not react this way. His questioning, at least overtly, took the form of constant reading about the possible biomedical causes of lupus. He was the mathematician, the scientist probing into causation and meaning on a physical, molecular level. He never blamed God, because, unlike my mother, he did not believe in God as a being who takes part in daily human life and can therefore be blamed for our misfortunes.

My friend Teresa reacted very differently. On the Christmas card she sent me, she wrote, "You know, Melissa, though you're having such a tough time with life right now, it's great that you can still smile and laugh through it. That's a tremendous inspiration to me. No one knows why some people suffer more than others, but there's a reason for everything, though only Jesus might know it. Keep strong, Melissa. I love you!" Though my experiences caused her to question why suffering exists, her faith that it has a purpose in God's plan did not waver. Her belief in God was an elemental part of her identity. She wanted to share some of that faith and love with me. When I read the letter, I remembered Kim.

Minh expressed her anger over the unfairness of my illness. She wrote to me that my experiences had caused her to examine her life.

I must admit that all your symptoms blew me away at first and made me wonder why I had been so concerned with my minuscule problems. You're so right to say that many things in life are more important than grades or a run in your panty hose. I came to appreciate my own health through this miserable cold. But the big difference is that I got over my cold. I'm very angry for you Melissa, because it seems so unfair. I have many friends that are all tied up in petty things, and I want to shake them all and make them see the light. I'm so tempted to thrust your letter in their face and say "Read this!" I'm sure it would shock them all into seeing things in a new perspective like it did for me.

Some chose not to ask the questions of meaning, because they could not bear to do so. For Bubbe Pearl and Zaide, my having a chronic illness made no sense. It violated a natural order. I was young; I had done nothing to deserve this. Besides, they loved me too much to believe that I could possibly be suffering from a chronic disease; therefore, to them, it could not be chronic. They believed that an instant cure lay within our immediate reach.

S pring became summer, and I came back to Maryland. My parents, especially my mother, had been eagerly awaiting my return to the nest, so they could take me under their wing and heal me. As my mother informed my brother, "Melissa is ours for the summer and I'm going to make her well whether she wants that or not." I let them "have me" for the summer. I felt that I had proved my point by staying at Laurel the entire year. Besides, I was too weak and ill to fight them anymore.

Mom watched over me to make sure that I rested. She fed me organic foods and vitamins. She insisted that I visit a nontraditional physician as well as various other traditional specialists, including a urologist, a gastroenterologist, and my endocrinologist, who had treated my slow thyroid since I was thirteen.

I also paid weekly visits to a physical therapist my mother found for me. In Kathleen Johnson, I found a health-care professional who was both dedicated and talented. She had a way of setting people at ease, with her words but mostly through her skilled and sensitive touch. On the first visit, she conducted a standard assessment of the range of motion in my joints and my muscle strength. Then treatment began. She brought me relief, but unfortunately, the lessening of pain and increased mobility did not last longer than a few hours after treatment.

As part of our sessions, Kathleen would ask me to walk up and down the halls so she could study my gait. She observed that I was throwing my right foot out to the right and slapping it down. I told Kathleen that I frequently caught my toes in sidewalk pavements. My mother had noticed the same movement pattern. It became most obvious to her, she said, when the entire family, grandparents included, were walking up a hill to an open-air theater. She saw how I was awkwardly dragging along behind everyone. Even Bubbe Pearl, who was seventy at the time, quickly outdistanced me, moving with far more agility than I.

After a few months of working with me, Kathleen had become quite concerned. She felt that the arthritis was severe enough to limit what she could do to help me. Also, at that point, she was worried that the abnormalities in my gait were caused by more than just arthritis. She wondered if my nervous system had become involved. She asked if she could speak with my rheumatologist, and I gave my permission. But according to Kathleen, Dr. Kostos was dismissive of her and her assessment of my condition. "Melissa's just suffering from arthritis and fatigue," he responded.

Several weeks later, I returned to Philadelphia to see Dr. Kostos. My sedimentation rate continued to be high, my ANA titer elevated. I also had mild high blood pressure. We talked about the use of oral steroids. Treatment for lupus can be conceived of as a pyramid. At its base are the least aggressive treatments, and at its peak the most powerful. As the disease increases in severity, the medications are chosen from higher up in the pyramid. The pyramid is composed of four basic levels. At the bottom are the NSAIDs. As one climbs the pyramid, one finds the antimalarials, then the steroids. The immunosuppressants, originally developed for cancer patients, occupy the summit. The pyramid, however, does not at all precisely dictate which regimens should be used for an individual at a given time. Treatment for lupus is highly variable and individual; what works for one patient might not be useful for another.

I had been unable to tolerate any of the NSAIDs. I was still taking Plaquenil, an antimalarial, but to little effect. However, Dr. Kostos adamantly refused to prescribe a steroid regimen. He explained his decision by telling me about a former patient, a young woman my age who also went to Laurel. He had treated her with prednisone. This patient felt so frustrated by the weight gain, the moon face, the facial hair, and the mood swings that are common side effects of steroids that she suddenly stopped taking them. She had been on a steroid regimen for a long time, so her adrenal glands had stopped functioning and could no longer produce cortisone (a necessary hormone) on their own. She died. I had my own fears about steroids. I was not eager to begin a steroid regimen, so I did not disagree. But I should have realized the flaw in his argument. He was speaking of another person, not making a medical judgment based on me or my own case. He was allowing his past painful experience with this one patient to overly determine how he should treat me.

The weeks wore on, filled with doctor's appointments and tests, all to no avail. Though none of the doctors I visited was able to stop the progression of the disease, some very important healing did take place, largely through the kind and wise ministrations of Evelyn McFadden. She was a psychologist recommended to me by my physical therapist. Evelyn McFadden specialized in treating people with chronic illnesses. One day, Kathleen handed me Evelyn McFadden's card. Kathleen said, "I'm not saying you need to go. But you're dealing with so much right now, and sometimes it helps to talk to someone—a person who isn't a friend or family member. And Evelyn is a wonderful therapist."

Eventually I did go to Evelyn McFadden. I arrived a bit early and waited with trepidation. I felt ashamed. I told myself that I should be able to handle this illness on my own without seeking professional help. Not only was my body diseased, but now I was also showing weakness of spirit. I should be facing my illness bravely, fearlessly, and now I had failed. Also, Dr. Smith's words rang in my ears. Had I proven her right? But despite my insecurities, I knew that my coming to Evelyn McFadden had nothing to do with Dr. Smith's suggestion that I seek psychologic counseling. I was not there to be treated for a psychosomatic disease. I just needed some help in coping with my chronic illness. I wanted to unburden myself to someone who was not directly involved in my life and speak openly to a person I did not have to protect. Also, I had been so fiercely focused in school that I had put many of my concerns and fears aside. Now that I was no longer in school and was spending so much of my time in the world of ill health, all the issues I had pushed to the background had leaped forward. I needed to sort them out. I was ready.

Evelyn, as she later asked me to call her, opened the door to her office and escorted another patient out. With her flaming red hair, pure white skin, and sapphire eyes, Evelyn was a striking woman. She was tall, about five feet eight, and slim. Her dress, a flowing African print, was stylish and slightly exotic. Her manner was warm as she welcomed me into her office.

My conceptions of mental health professionals had come mainly from movies and novels. I expected to lie down on a couch while a severe, remote psychologist or psychiatrist sat in an authoritarian position above me. But Evelyn invited me to sit down in one of the overstuffed, comfortable chairs. She sat down opposite me in an identical chair. There was a couch in the office, but I never made use of it. The setting was informal, soothing, and inviting.

The walls were painted peach, and plants graced the windowsill. There was a New Mexican touch to the decor of the room. On her wall hung several striking paintings. One depicted a pueblo with a Native American woman sitting in front. The woman was old, her broad face wrinkled by the sun, her figure stooped, most of her teeth missing. But she smiled as she held a fat, laughing, dark-haired, brown-eyed baby in her lap. In her delight in the child, she became beautiful. When I looked at the picture, I wanted to smile. I also enjoyed Evelyn's painting of a rock formation, its jutting tan-and-ocher edges set on fire by the rising sun. The artist did not see the desert as barren, arid. Through his eyes, the desert became a place of spectacular color, immense space, and freedom. When I looked at the office, I saw the vitality of its occupant. I thought to myself, "I have come to the right place."

I visited her once a week. She never judged me, only guided me to valuable insights that brought me some peace. I adopted a different attitude about romantic relationships. Instead of being discouraged by Carlos's inability to handle the illness and assuming that most men would have the same difficulty, I decided that I was not being fair to myself or to the men I was dating. I needed to be more open and give the man a chance. I also concluded that, in a way, I am lucky. After all, I know that the man who falls in love with me loves me for who I am despite my limitations. And are we not all limited in some way?

Most important, Evelyn helped me to understand that I could accept assistance from others without diminishment of self, because I could still help others, even if not as I had before. Maybe I could not walk far out of my way on campus to run an errand for a friend or perform all kinds of other favors that involved too much physical strain. But when I thought about the previous school year, I realized that because I stayed mostly on the first floor, my friends usually came down to visit me instead of the other way around. Gradually my room became a center where my friends could relax and unburden themselves. After complaining about her current boyfriend and asking my advice, one friend teased, "Melissa, you should hang out a shingle—'Melissa's Counseling Services.'" I was the resident editor who critiqued papers. There was always my writing, a way of connecting myself to others. I could still enjoy rich, full relationships that included giving and receiving on both sides. Possessing the knowledge that I could contribute to others was of paramount importance to me. I could still be the kind of person I respected. I could let go of the shame I had been carrying with me these past nine months. I also felt more secure; I no longer feared that people would abandon me.

Though this was a harder lesson for me to grasp, I learned how essential it was for others in my life to be able to help me. Their need to give was as deep as mine. They, too, felt powerless when confronted by my illness.

They only felt more frustrated and helpless when, in my efforts to shield them and to maintain my independence, I would not confide in them or accept their offers of assistance.

Last of all, I came to terms with the basic fact that I did need some help, because I could not do everything I had done before, no matter how hard I tried. Acceptance of my physical limitations was the hardest lesson for me, one I had not entirely mastered by the end of the time I spent with Evelyn. Though I know that I will probably pay a price, even now, in work and in play, I sometimes find it difficult to avoid overexerting myself. But overall, I learned more easily to balance my needs for independence, my family's and my friends' desire to help me, and the physical limitations imposed by my illness.

At the end of the summer, I dreamt that I stood before a lake whose waters were blue-black and churning. The sky hung thunderously overhead while I waited helplessly on the shore. Then from the depths of me the words came hurtling up, "I'm afraid!" It was as if the words possessed a shape and a force. But once they reached the open air, they disintegrated and fell like a soft rain upon me and the waters. Then, to my surprise, the lake stilled and the sky lightened. I woke with the words still on my lips. But what I felt was not fear but an immense relief and calm. A terrible weight had been lifted.

Now, as I look back, I realize how essential that summer was in my reaching some kind of initial acceptance of the disease. I also understand that those basic struggles—overcoming my shame about needing and asking for help, conquering my fear of being abandoned by others, attempting to keep my self-respect, independence, and identity—never ended. For me, they are part of the wolf and always will be. But I also know that, today, though I continue to fight many of the same battles, I act out of a solid foundation of strength and confidence that I did not possess at the beginning.

My own emotional healing and coming to terms with my illness rippled out to touch my family and friends. Because I was truly beginning to accept my illness, my parents and I were able to really discuss how we felt about everything that had happened over the past year. My father and I resolved our differences after several heartfelt conversations in which I convinced him that I must manage my own illness and that I would be capable of doing so. Recognizing that being home surrounded by his and my mother's love was no cure, and confident that I could handle my illness, he felt able to let me go back to school in September.

My mother finally talked about the terrible, corrosive guilt that she had been harboring. She felt that she had caused my disease in some way. Though lupus can be considered a genetic disorder, the disease is not seen to be directly inherited. Each parent must contribute genes to create a predisposition for the illness, but the mechanisms behind the activation of those genes remain unknown. My mother *knew* that she had given me half of the lupus genes. Her sense of responsibility was further compounded by the mystery surrounding the triggering of the disease. She wondered if she had committed some sins of commission or omission while I was growing up, mistakes that had set off the lupus. Perhaps she had not fed me the proper foods, or maybe she had inadvertently exposed me to something harmful.

But then my mother had her own dream, which she shared with me one afternoon. "In my dream, I was making my way through a vast jungle, searching for the famous witch doctor. I was hoping he could tell me how to cure you. I finally met him in a clearing. He was covered with white beads that shone against his black skin. He gestured for me to sit down beside him. I remember looking into those deep brown eyes and thinking that he knew why I had come and that he understood my pain. I asked him, 'How can I cure my daughter?' He gazed at me thoughtfully, but he never spoke a word out loud. Then a voice began to speak in my head. It said, 'You cannot cure your daughter. Your job is not to cure her. But you can help her by giving her love and support when she needs you, and space and freedom too.' But I wanted to know how exactly to do that. The voice told me that it couldn't answer that question for me; I would have to figure it out for myself. After that, the witch doctor got up, placed a strand of his beads around my neck, and disappeared into the jungle."

By the end of the summer, my mother became less protective and obsessive about finding a cure. When it came time for me to return to Laurel, like my father, she was ready to let me go.

> She sees me walk with unsteady gait,
> grown child who has forgotten the steps.
> It brings to her mind days long ago
> when she held out her hands
> watched me totter toward her
> on chubby legs used to crawling.
> When I arrived in her arms

crowing with pride,
she crooned to me with a mother's promise,
"I will keep you safe always, my life upon it."
Now my legs that had grown strong and sturdy
stumble, clumsy and slow on their path.
She calls to me, her voice heavy
with the weight of her broken oath,
"Come into my arms
that can heal and protect you"
and hopes to make the impossible true.
But the circle of her embrace
does not hold my life
only the love sustaining me
in my journey forward. I pull away.
In anguish she feels her empty arms fall to her side,
but then as she follows me with her gaze,
she sees her child grown,
realizing she has kept a mother's only promise,
the certainty of her love and the uncertainty of life.
I turn to her and smile;
we are joined together
healed.

The summer was a time of healing and deepening relationships. Bubbe Pearl and Zaide came to recognize the reality of the lupus. My grandfather no longer demanded whether or not I was cured yet. They did not advise me to solve my health problems by becoming more physically active or just cheering up. I no longer cringed from their well-meaning but hurtful comments. We were able to enjoy more open conversations about the illness. Today they are two of the most loyal members in my support system. When I need advice and comfort, I call them, and I am always received with love and understanding.

My growing acceptance of my illness also allowed me to communicate more openly with my friends. Before I returned to school, I wrote to Jessica, Mary, and Teresa. I explained that I would need to rely on them a bit more than I had before for emotional and practical support. I said that we had all been denying the reality of my illness to a certain extent, but this would need to change for me to cope successfully at school. Jessica replied,

You really hit the nail on the head when you said that we all have to accept your illness. I realize that you have lupus, but it is quite another matter to comprehend that you can't do certain things and you are not always feeling your perky self. I guess I felt if I believed hard enough you would be able to do everything you could freshman year. It's weird to write that because I'd convinced myself that I was handling the lupus better than most. Anyway, I want you to feel free to talk to me anytime about what you're going through. And promise me you will *immediately* notify me when I'm not being understanding or realistic. This may be hard to do, but I want to be a help not a hindrance.

Teresa and Mary were equally supportive in their letters.

Though I was working toward building relationships in which I could be honest about my illness, I also learned that not everyone would be able to accept my illness and be able to support me in that respect, no matter how many times I tried to discuss it. To this day, one of my relatives does not comprehend the illness and its effect on my life. I learned to accept such people as they were, and I hoped they would do the same for me. And I treasured even more those understanding people with whom I could be completely candid.

9

Blue Shimmering Waters

Fall 1989

EASED IN spirit if not in body, I returned to school. The fall of 1989 was an exciting academic semester. I found a professor who became both my mentor and friend. During a lifetime, everyone recognizes some person, event, or decision to be life altering. The decision to sign up for Dr. Esther Stein's course was a life changing moment for me. The class, "The Sociology of Bioethics" was not one I had heard of, and I was not even familiar with the term "bioethics." But the course description sounded intriguing, and by that time, because of my personal experiences, I was developing an intellectual interest in the medical world. Each semester I tried to take a course outside the English department and the other departments I usually haunted. Since I had not yet ventured into sociology, I thought I would give it a try.

When Dr. Stein entered the classroom that first day of the seminar, my first impression was of a woman in her late fifties or possibly early sixties with thick, wavy gray hair that just brushed the top of her collar. Her eyes were gray-blue, lively, and warm; later I learned how keenly she used them to observe the world around her. I immediately noticed how petite she was, tiny-boned almost to the point of fragility. She walked with a slight limp. But as she lectured, her articulateness, her stunning intelligence, and her breadth of knowledge became her most obvious characteristics, not any seeming physical frailty.

The class was conducted as a seminar. I found the topics—including transplantation, the artificial heart, abortion, and surrogate motherhood— fascinating. We were assigned one long term paper on a topic of our choice.

Dr. Stein and I met several times to talk about my paper, "Managing Chronic Illness as a Young Adult." She was enthusiastic about my research. I talked to her about some of my illness experiences, because they were material for my paper. We also spoke about my classes, the other class I was taking that semester, the classes I would take next term, and my plans for the future.

So began our lasting relationship. In Esther I have come to know a genuine Renaissance scholar whose interests range across the arts and sciences. I also discovered that her strength encompasses that of the spiritual as well as the mind. She is devoted to teaching, but her conception of her role as professor extends beyond imparting information about a particular subject. She is mentor and friend to many, generously offering her gentle guidance, wise advice, and constant support.

It is always hard to predict what might or might not happen if certain events do not take place. I cannot be sure, but I really do not think I would have taken Esther's course if I had not become ill. My interest in medical issues, at least in the beginning, stemmed directly from my own experiences. So I believe that because of the lupus, I met Esther. In her and in our many endeavors together, I am reminded that lupus has brought me a rare gift, even through pain.

Throughout the fall semester, I also enjoyed a more relaxed and open relationship with my friends at school. No longer was lupus the dreaded L-word. I learned that asking for help from my friends became easier by keeping in mind who would be most appropriate for each task. Teresa was the best person to accompany me to the emergency room. Perhaps because her mother is a nurse, the hospital is not such an intimidating place to Teresa. Because Mary passes out at the sight of blood, I kept her away from the hospital. But she loves to shop, so it was no problem for her to pick up a few things at the drugstore or the grocery. Jessica never minded running any errands on campus. I tried to spread out my requests evenly so that no one in my support system would be overburdened.

At the end of the semester, I shared my paper "Managing Chronic Illness as a Young Adult" with Jessica, Mary, and Teresa. Another good friend of ours, Mark, saw them reading the paper and asked if he might read it as well. After he finished he came to me and said, "Thank you so much for letting me read this. It explains a lot. I've been feeling upset these past months because you weren't saying anything about the lupus. I thought you were talking to other people, but for whatever reasons, you felt that you couldn't talk to me. It seemed that our friendship didn't mean much to you. I didn't know how I should bring up the subject."

I was shocked. Precisely because I cared about him and our friendship, I had been trying to shield him from my disease. But I had only hurt him. My paper opened the door to many honest discussions and a more intimate friendship. After graduation, he called to tell me that he was gay. He said that he was able to confide in me because I had trusted him with my illness. He knew I would not judge him or run away. We could accept each other as we were.

Though it was a positive time for nourishing mind and soul, it was also a time of unrelenting disease. The fatigue and fevers were unremitting. I suffered from frequent infections—bladder and sinus infections, flus, and colds. Infections aggravated my lupus symptoms. My rheumatologist told me that the stomach problems plaguing me were caused by serositis of the abdomen, an inflammation of the membranes lining the abdomen.

I was also having increasing difficulty using my hands. It became even harder to keep objects in my shaky grasp, and I lost more sensation in my hands. Completing basic tasks were increasingly frustrating problems to be solved. Using silverware, dialing a phone, and putting my keys in my front door all became difficult. Sometimes I had to dial a number five or six times before I got it right.

Throughout that fall, the physical therapist who was treating me at school discovered that the weakness in my neck, leg, and arm muscles was increasing. Even a simple task such as washing my hair turned into a painful, exhausting chore. Each time I finished showering, my arms and hands ached so badly that I would resolve to cut my hair short so that it would be easier to care for. But I could not do it. My long curls had always been part of what made me feel feminine and pretty. So I kept my hair long in my attempt to keep alive some sense of myself as an attractive young woman.

Moving around became more of a challenge as the abnormalities in my gait became more pronounced. When I walked—slowly, stiffly, not always certain of my balance—I was slapping my right foot down, dragging it along with me as if it were an ineptly attached appendage. My rheumatologist continued to assert that my gait and general weakness were the result of arthritis and fatigue, and that I would just have to live with it.

As well as the headaches, I was also experiencing what I called "fuzzyheadedness." I was just not as clear-minded or alert as usual, my memory was not as sharp, and I was having trouble concentrating. This symptom frightened me the most, because my mind was *me*. My being able to stay in school, to pursue my career, ultimately depended on my ability to think.

As the Christmas vacation neared, my family and I discussed our plans to take a cruise to the Caribbean. We had taken such a cruise the previous December, before I had become ill, and I longed to be on board ship again, exploring the waters of the clear, gentle Caribbean Sea. I wanted to roam the colorful islands, calling on different ports this time. Though a cruise is probably the least strenuous kind of vacation, my parents were quite concerned that I was not well enough to go. But Dr. Kostos gave his approval for the trip.

Dr. Kostos had never placed any real limitations on my activities. I was permitted to do whatever I could. In the past few fall months, as my symptoms grew worse, he had repeatedly told me that I just had to learn to live with my problems. There were no other options. I trusted his opinion and assessment of the situation. Besides, the abnormal had become my normal. Within this context, my primary question became "How can I continue to function in this physical state and do the things that are most important to me?" I learned that I had extensive reserves, and I drew upon them over and over to complete my schoolwork and participate in social activities. I also found that I had a high threshold for pain and a talent for distracting myself from it in order to do and be.

I could escape pain by becoming absorbed in the conversation of friends and family. My studies drew me in as well, offering me a place of refuge. Visualization and fantasy were two very powerful weapons I often used. They were particularly helpful when I walked any distance, an activity the arthritis made excruciating. I often thought of the Hans Christian Andersen fairy tale in which the mermaid leaves her sea home to marry a prince. To live on dry land, she must give up her tail for legs, and when she walks, it is as if a thousand knives pierce her feet. Sometimes I would think bitterly that at least the mermaid won her prince and true love in return for her pain. I had struck no such bargain. But most of the time, my thoughts were not so gloomy. I made my way around the city and the campus, overcoming my pain and fatigue by disappearing into fantasy. As I spun out detailed stories, my legs kept moving, keeping rhythm with my imagination. Picturing winning the Pulitzer prize for my first novel usually carried me a good six or seven blocks!

Most of the time, I functioned astoundingly well considering the physical shape I was in. But sometimes the pain overwhelmed me, and I could not continue in my daily routine. Then I usually turned to music, one of my strongest defenses against pain. Sweet jazz works best for me—Nat King Cole or Louis Armstrong.

In the music pain cannot find me. As the sound of the sax fills my being, I slip into another world, one created by the music and me. I am in a jazz club, small, intimate, sensual. Candles flicker on the tiny round tables surrounding the smooth, wooden dance floor, which is the color of poured honey. And I dance. Always in the arms of a man whose face I cannot see, but I feel his arms around me as we sway gracefully to the music. I am loved and protected. I feel beautiful in my dress of red silk and my elegant high heels. There is no illness, no pain. I move with lightness and freedom, warmed by the dancing and the wine. When I leave my jazz club, I am refreshed; the pain is eased.

So, this is how, even in my deteriorating state, I was able to set off on the voyage. I gave myself over to the joys of traveling and vacation, determined that the lupus would not rob me of my pleasure in this trip. I had always greatly enjoyed swimming and had been regularly swimming at the school gym. Exercising in the water provided some relief for the arthritis. So it is not surprising that my favorite part of the cruise was going snorkeling. At the Grand Caymans, a group of us went out in a small boat. The captain stopped at scenic spots where there was either a shipwreck, an abundance of tropical fish, or an especially beautiful coral reef. Though I had always been entranced by watching the sea, I loved becoming a part of it in this way and learning some of the secrets it kept hidden beneath its surface.

Unfortunately, my delight in the vacation did not have the power to stop my symptoms. By the end of the cruise I was feeling worse than when I had come on board. I think the proverbial last straw was a tour of the historic fort in San Juan. The tropical sun beat down upon our heads, and there was no cover. By the time we got back to the ship, I had a sunburn. From then on, I felt increasingly ill.

When family members and I tell the story of the crippling lupus flare that followed, we always begin with that excursion to San Juan. We cannot say with any certainty that if I had avoided that tour, I would have prevented the flare that became tattooed in all of our memories. After all, I had been increasingly symptomatic for months. But the stories we tell about the events in our lives must begin somewhere, and in choosing that place to start, we are organizing the story, giving events causes. And that is what my family and I do when we give an account of that terrible flare; we are explaining it to ourselves. Like everyone who faces a mysterious disease, my family and I need to create some kind of order out of randomness. We were, and still are, constantly faced with the guessing game of trying to pinpoint what triggers the disease. How does it become active? If we could know, we could gain some control over it and not be completely at its mercy.

Weak and exhausted, I did return to school for the spring term. In a few days, I was unable to hold down liquids. All my symptoms quickly became more severe, including intense lower back pain and headaches. By that time, I had no reserves left. Visualization and distraction techniques were not going to be enough to allow me to function.

My aunt Beth knew what was happening and was extremely concerned. She spoke to my mother and received strict instructions to take me to the emergency room. Under duress, too weak to argue, I went.

So began the nightmare.

10

Betrayals in the Desert

January 1990—May 1990

I T WAS early evening when we entered the emergency room of the
inner-city hospital. As we opened the glass doors, we found ourselves
in a place harshly, unrelentingly lit by fluorescents that caught the
people and objects in a pitiless glare. The chairs, blindingly bright orange
and dull institutional green, were vinyl and plastic and stood on a tile floor
of uncertain color, probably once white, now an indeterminate gray. A
homeless person, his skin the color of ashes, sat in one corner, rocking,
muttering, moaning, and occasionally looking up to view the other people
in the room with suspicion. The chairs to the left, right, and front of him
were vacant. Everyone in the room took care not to meet his gaze.

I registered, then settled down to begin the long wait to be seen by a
physician. A few minutes later, my aunt and I heard yelling, screaming, and
cursing. Two cops walked into the ER. One cop was pushing a wheelchair
which held a man whose wrists were handcuffed to the chair. The man
jerked and twisted his body, straining with the effort of trying to escape the
wheelchair and the cuffs. As the cops brought the chair toward me on their
way to the examining rooms, I realized that the man in the wheelchair
might only be a teenager. It was difficult to determine his age because of his
garish, thick layers of makeup, which included foundation and eye shadow.
Blood painted his face and shaved head and dotted the sleeves of his cheap
black leather jacket. The cops were quite casual in their attitude, even
bored, as if they had seen this before and would again.

Like most people in today's society, I had been exposed to graphic
crime and violence through Hollywood and the news media. But I was still

not prepared for this situation. I heard the cops nonchalantly tell the doctors that the young man was a strung-out junkie who had been involved in a gang fight. I was not distanced from what was going on, not watching television or reading the paper in the comfort and security of my own home. This was happening a few feet away from me. I could feel this man's malice and hatred, a consuming emotion that washed over the room in corrosive waves. The policemen rolled him back to be treated immediately. We in the waiting room could hear the man's continued bellows and the attempts of the doctors to soothe him while they stitched his wounds. We also heard the clatter of instruments falling to the floor and the threats of the cops if the prisoner did not behave. I wondered how this man or boy had become an addict. What was his life like? What fed such rage? Was there any hope for him?

My aunt and I continued to wait. A woman came to sit beside us. She looked to be in her mid-forties, well-groomed, and expensively dressed. In a soft, pleasant voice she struck up a conversation. She seemed to be a welcome reminder of the normal world I had left outside the ER doors. Eventually, she started to tell us her troubles, and we felt quite sorry for her. Then she assured us that everything would be all right because the aliens, who were her real family, were coming to take her back to her home planet any day now. The woman described her world, Zeptar, in great detail. As she went on, her eyes took on a glazed, faraway look, and her voice trembled. She seemed as lost and troubled as the junkie or the homeless person surrounded by all the empty chairs.

After a few hours, we were taken back to the examining rooms. The nurse gave me a gown to change into and instructed me to lay on the gurney which was about as soft as a sidewalk. She told me that the doctor would be in soon, and a frazzled intern did eventually arrive. After taking a history and establishing that the problems bringing me to the ER were mainly gastric, including nausea, uncontrolled vomiting, abdominal pain, and diarrhea, he began his physical exam. First he tried to take my blood pressure while I was lying down, sitting up, and standing up. The blood pressure should be stable from one position to the other; if not, this indicates dehydration. He had difficulty getting a reading while I was standing up because the ER was so noisy. I was feeling extremely faint, dizzy, and nauseous. When I politely but firmly tried to tell the intern that I was really feeling nauseous and needed to lie down, he ignored me and continued to listen for the pressure. Finally I could hold out no more. I vomited all over his shoes.

The intern decided it would be wise to give me medication to stop the vomiting and to hydrate me. He gave me a shot of an extremely powerful anti-emetic drug that is used to prevent vomiting while a patient is undergoing surgery, then began IV fluids. A few minutes after the drug was administered, I developed a bizarre allergic reaction. I felt as if my tongue had swollen to huge proportions. I could not speak normally; it was like talking with marbles in my mouth. I became completely irrational and started to throw myself from side to side on the gurney. In a nasty tone of voice, I said to my aunt, "I hate you. It's all your fault we're here. I'm leaving. I want to see that doctor, because I'm signing myself out AMA [against medical advice]." She found the doctor, who gave me a shot of cogentin, a drug that countered the psychomotor response I was having, and the allergic reaction subsided.

The intern convinced me to stay. After he had hydrated me to his satisfaction and drawn blood to run various tests, he called my rheumatologist. Dr. Kostos said that I should be discharged and come to see him in his office the following day.

It was past one in the morning when we left the hospital. My aunt told me to wait for her inside the entryway while she brought the car. I was too tired to walk to the lot located only a block away. After I got into the car, I saw that she had been crying. She burst out, "You still love me, don't you? You're not angry at me for bringing you here?" I replied, "Of course not, that was the drugs talking, not me. You know I love you." She seemed reassured and less anxious, but after that we spoke little, both of us exhausted beyond speech.

My aunt worked in another hospital close by, and my dorm was only a few miles away from the ER. Yet that night, all was strange and unfamiliar to us. In confusion, we rode down empty city streets that seemed beseiged by a heavy darkness against which the streetlights battled with little success. Lost, we wandered the city, even going the wrong way down a one-way street. Time became distorted; it felt as if we had been on the road for hours, our path blocked at every turn. Finally, almost an hour later, we did find my dorm. When I arrived home, I immediately stumbled into bed, falling into a deep but troubled sleep, my dreams filled with disturbing, disjointed memories of my visit to the ER and vague apprehensions of what tomorrow's appointment might bring.

When I met with him the next morning, Dr. Kostos decided to admit me to the hospital that day in order to treat the lupus flare. The two and a half weeks that followed are mostly a blur in my memory—a hazy expanse broken only by a few clear and vivid images and scenes. Both the medications I was given and the disease dulled my mind. But I also think that it has been a gift of memory to let that time become misted over, not lost or buried, but also not sharply remembered. To reconstruct events I have had to rely heavily on doctor's records, journal entries written after I was discharged, and interviews with family and friends.

I do remember my hospital room, perhaps because I rarely left it. The semiprivate room was small and cramped, barely large enough for two beds, two nightstands, two bed tables, and necessary equipment like IV poles or bedside commodes. The lack of space made maneuvering in the room a challenge for patients, staff, and family. The room was dim and filthy with accumulated grime. On the wall above my bed was an old bloodstain. In color and cleanliness the tile floor was a replica of the one in the ER. Dustballs grew and multiplied underneath the bed and in the corners. Trashcans overflowed. Housekeeping did not come often, and when they did, their efforts were half-hearted.

Into this room came the medical teams, appearing and disappearing like flocks of white gulls, peering at me with curious eyes. I was treated by three different teams: rheumatology, gastroenterology, and internal medicine. In order to diagnose my stomach problems, the gastroenterology team ordered an upper GI. At this point, I was unable to even hold down water, yet the gastroenterologists requested a test that requires swallowing large amounts of a thick barium solution. Predictably, I vomited the barium all over myself and the x-ray table.

After performing an upper endoscopy, in which a scope is passed down the throat into the stomach, the gastroenterologists concluded that I had gastritis (inflammation of the stomach) and esophageal reflux (regurgitation of the stomach contents). Dr. Kostos cited serositis of the abdomen as the cause of my gastric symptoms. Blood work showed that I was malnourished and dehydrated. A bone scan revealed inflammation in all the major joints. My sed rate and ANA titer continued to be elevated.

A few days after I was admitted, the initial testing having been completed, I was given IV pulse steroids. My physician admitted that the treatment had not been that effective for me in the past. However, it would not harm me, and he needed to prescribe a drug regimen to justify keeping me in the hospital in the eyes of the hospital board. I was kept hydrated and given a medicine to combat the continual nausea and vomiting. Unfortunately, the medicine did nothing but make me extremely drowsy.

My strength ebbed with each passing day, my steps in the hallway becoming more hesitant and slow. I began to fall when I walked or stood for any length of time. Even my hands and arms were weak. I reached a point when I could not pull myself up in bed or rise out of a chair without assistance. Eventually I required a bedside commode. The weakness was accompanied by a diminishing of sensation, from my waist down to my toes, as well as in my hands and arms. I had severe back pain. My family and I were told that my weakness resulted from deconditioning. In other words, I was out of shape because I was spending so much time in bed. "Even athletes become deconditioned within a few days of bed rest," Dr. Kostos said with a reassuring smile.

I also developed problems with my bladder. I would feel an intense urge to urinate, but when I tried, my bladder closed tight. When I was able to pass urine, the sensation was not normal. For about five days I was straight catheterized whenever I felt the need to urinate. A tube was inserted into my bladder in order to empty it. My physicians assumed, because I had a history of urinary-tract infections (UTIs), that my symptoms were the result of another UTI. But they could find no evidence of infection. A urologist was called in to consult but was unable to explain my symptoms. He did comment on the weakness in my legs, but no further mention of it was made by him or by the other physicians. Eventually the physicians did find a UTI. A few years later, other physicians told me that the UTI was actually introduced by the repeated straight catheterizations; the UTI was only a complication of medical intervention rather than the cause of my bladder problems.

In the days leading up to that last terrible night before discharge, I lived for the most part from moment to moment, neither thinking nor feeling deeply about what was happening to me. I needed all of my strength to cope with my physical pain and weakness. I did not possess the energy and mental clarity for much introspection, for worries about the ultimate course of my disease, or for questions and doubts about my recovery.

I have found that during my hospital stays, I slip into what I call my Scarlett O'Hara role, telling myself "I'll think about all that tomorrow." For me it has been an extremely effective way to get through the days spent in the hospital. After the crisis is over and I come home, tomorrow arrives. My protective calm shatters, and I am caught up in the aftermath of the hospital experiences. The hospital stays dramatically remind me of my vulnerability to this unpredictable disease. As I struggle to recover and adapt to any new disabilities, I mourn, looking backward to "my treasured past / Filled with beauty, joy and delight." When I turn my gaze forward, I see "Future's landscape blighted by disease." I finally turn toward the Present, yet all I can see is barren earth. But I take up my gardening tools again, toiling until I make my Present garden bloom once more.

So, at least until that final night, I do not remember feeling intense emotions about my condition or casting my mind ahead to all the uncertainties of my future. I do clearly recall the pain, discomfort, and disabling weakness. But what lives with equal power in my memory is the sense of my family's and friends' constant presence. Their unstinting gifts of friendship, love, support, and good wishes were continual and sustaining.

My memories of my parents are particularly distinct. In this acute period of my lupus I became like a child again, needing my parents' care. I relied completely on them. My mother and my father each took on different roles. Though my father's love for me is unbounded, his tolerance for hospitals is limited. The realities of my sickness and the hospital were too painful for him to bear. He became irritable and restless when he spent any extended amount of time in my room, so we often sent him on errands while my mom remained with me. In doing things for me, he could express his love and help me in a way that he could handle. When my father did stay with me, he usually slept. I still see him, a thick paperback, usually a spy novel or a thriller, laid across his lap. He would read for a few minutes and then flee into the forgetfulness of sleep.

My mother did not have this luxury for she was my nurse, physician, and advocate. She arrived early in the morning and stayed until at least nine or ten o'clock at night, sometimes later. Without her vigilance and attention, I do not know how I would have fared in that hospital. First of all, because the hospital nursing staff was too small to provide adequate care, my mother's role as a nurse was essential. I tried to minimize the number of times I pressed the call button. When I did signal for a nurse, I really needed one to come, but it was often twenty minutes or even a half hour before anyone responded. I still can remember the utter sense of helplessness, shame, and pain while I was waiting for a nurse to answer my call and catheterize me. I learned to push my call button at the first hint that my bladder was filling, so that the pressure pain might not reach an excruciating level.

When a nurse did arrive, she (sometimes he) would rush into my room, usually apologizing and explaining that she was attending to an emergency and that there were no other nurses covering the other patients. I was just fortunate that my mother was often able to take care of me herself. If I required the services of a nurse, she went out to the nurses' station, refusing to budge until a nurse could be located.

One of my roommates was not as lucky as I. No family or friends ever came to visit. She was completely dependent upon the nurses and her call button. Early one morning, before my family arrived, her IV pulled out, and she began to bleed profusely. This was dangerous because she was on a blood thinner. She put on her call button, but received no reply. She also asked me to press mine. Still no answer. At least fifteen minutes elapsed. I was too weak to get out of bed, and she was immobilized with a broken hip. As we watched helplessly, blood soaked the sheets, then the floor. Finally she said, "I'm from South Philly. We know how to make a lot of noise, and I'm gonna do just that." She started to yell. Even with that, it took another five or ten minutes before a nurse showed up.

Once a nurse was found, he or she often needed to consult with a physician in order to discuss what to do about the problem. However, communications between the physicians and nurses were anything but efficient. Many times I waited for hours while a nurse attempted to find a physician, then for hours more until the orders were carried out. My mother would advocate for me until the situation was resolved.

My mother brought supplies from home because the hospital was not fully stocked. She was asked to get several of my drugs at an outside pharmacy because the hospital did not carry them. The drugs were not unusual medications, and other hospitals in which I have stayed have not had any difficulties filling the prescriptions. When my back pain was at its worst, my nurse attempted to procure a heating pad and a layer of foam to make the mattress more comfortable, but these basic items were unavailable. She exclaimed angrily, "Nothing is ever here when you need it," then apologized for her outburst and suggested that my mom bring a heating pad from home.

As the nurses frequently apologized and explained the delays and the shortages, I sensed their own frustration. They were being asked to do their job within a disorganized system that provided far too little in the way of supplies and personnel. The result was considerably less than optimal care for patients and, from what I observed, much disgruntlement amongst the nurses.

My mom became a part of the medical team in other important ways. My medical care was fragmented; the various specialists did not seem to communicate with one another. My mother attempted to fill that vacuum by keeping the various medical teams or individual doctors informed about what the other teams or doctors had told us. She supervised the prescribing of medication and medical regimens. I was fortunate that she did so, because she discovered that one doctor had prescribed three times the dosage of one of my usual medications.

Because of her persistence, I finally received IV nutrition. She was particularly concerned about my malnutrition. She very firmly felt that if I were able to get nutrients into my system, I would become stronger; the persistent and overwhelming nausea might ease as well. But I could not hold down anything she tried to feed me by mouth, such as homemade chicken broth or tea with molasses in it. I particularly remember her bringing the jar of molasses every day for over a week. I see her carefully spooning the sweet, thick stuff into my tea, hoping to inject strength and health with each drop. But one day she lost hold of the jar while attempting to open it. The jar dropped to the floor, shattering into a dark-brown pool that glinted with shards of glass. Though Mom and housekeeping tried to clean up the mess, the floor stayed sticky until I left.

Soon after the molasses jar broke, my mother decided that we must find another way for me to receive some nutrition. The physicians had been unable to offer any suggestions. Frustrated, my mother decided to investigate the problem herself by talking with the nurses. She inquired, "Isn't there any way of giving her some kind of nutrition through the IV?" Eventually a nurse told her about PPN, peripheral parenteral nutrition. PPN is an IV solution that contains a mixture of vitamins, minerals, proteins, and carbohydrates. My mother immediately demanded to see my rheumatologist and the gastroenterologist and insisted that they administer PPN. They agreed that it was a good idea. Within a few days of receiving PPN, my nausea and vomiting subsided.

Once the nausea and vomiting were under control, I was able to tolerate clear liquids, then a soft diet. I had been given antibiotics for the bladder infection, but the sensation while urinating was still not normal. Nor had I regained any of the sensation I had lost—in the lower half of my body, from the waist down; in my hands; and in my arms. I was as weak as before, and I continued to fall. However, because the gastric problems for which I had been admitted had been successfully treated, Dr. Kostos decided that I was ready to be discharged.

A resident brought me the paperwork to make my release official. He lingered in the room as I prepared to leave. I got out of bed and stood up. Before I knew what was happening, I had landed in a crumpled heap on the floor. I was not hurt, and by this time, I was not exactly surprised, though not pleased, to find myself on the floor. The resident was a tall man, over six feet, with the broad shoulders and muscular build of a football player. In one smooth motion he scooped me up and put me back into bed. Then he called Dr. Kostos.

It was about five o'clock. My roommate had been discharged earlier. The sun was setting, bleeding the light from the room. All was unusually quiet. Little noise or activity filtered in from the hallways, for the evening visitors had not yet arrived. I was lying in bed when Dr. Kostos entered.

In a voice devoid of emotion, he ordered, "Out of bed. On your feet." With difficulty, I was able to stand, but after a few seconds, I fell. Motionless, he stared down at me. Mom was beside him. She moved forward to help me, but he put his hand on her arm to restrain her. "You can get up, Melissa. Pick yourself up off the floor," he commanded. As I lay there, he towered over me, a chilling figure in white. I did not feel any anger coming from him, only a complete detachment and withdrawal that hit me like an icy blast. My mother was not coming to my aid either and had not spoken. I had not seen her make a move to come toward me, and I did not notice his holding her back. She told me later that she was frozen in shocked disbelief, watching the scene unfold as if she were standing outside herself. All I knew at that moment was how I felt—abandoned, humiliated, alone in my weakness.

I scrabbled feebly on the dirty tile, attempting to pull myself up by grasping the siderails of the bed. If Dr. Kostos, in whom I had so trusted and believed, said that there was no reason why I should not be able to get up, then it must be true. But I could not stand. I was very weak, but my inability to get up resulted from more than that. I willed the legs to move, the hands to clasp the bed railing, but it was as if my limbs had forgotten how to carry out my orders. I had not the faintest idea of how to go about movements I had always done naturally.

The minutes ticked by, slowly, silently. Sweat trickled down my face as I struggled with a body that would not obey me. It was becoming more obvious, at least to me, that I could not get myself off the ground. Yet Dr. Kostos did not move to assist me. Why? Why were my body and my physician betraying me this way?

Finally I was able to grab the handrails and pull myself to a sitting position. Dr. Kostos hauled me to my feet. Barely looking at me, he said I could stay one more night in the hospital. Then I would be sent home. With those few words, he disappeared, leaving me in the darkened room.

Pain blazes through me
in crimson flickering flames.
When will I ever be free
of the fire again?

I used to dance and play
under a beneficent sky.
Parents kept all harm at bay;
all that was good was mine.

But now disease grips my life
with fangs and claws of steel.
Thank God in all this strife
the doctor is here to heal!

Yet as disease rips away
the life I used to know,
my faith in doctors turns so gray;
my disillusionment only grows.

I can fight the enemy
with head held high and proud.
For illness attacks impartially—
with vengeance unendowed.

But the doctor's evil
is so hard to fight,
for that kind of devil
hides in a trusted coat of white.

Held in my mother's arms, I wept for the first time since I had entered the hospital. I cried for the events of that night and for all that had happened in the past few weeks. I shed tears for the immediate future that was shadowed with frightening uncertainty. I was worried about how I could possibly manage at home in my weakened condition. I could not perform any basic tasks without special equipment and/or someone's assistance. I had a built-up commode. I could not bathe, dress, or feed myself without help. I could not walk without falling. I could not manage steps. When I thought of all that, I was frightened of leaving the hospital, as horrifying as it had been. I was not being discharged with any follow-up services. In his discharge instructions, Dr. Kostos asked only that I make an appointment

to see him in a few weeks. The next morning I left the hospital, returning to Maryland with my parents. As I got out of the bed, all my limbs
were tensed in fear. When I landed safely, if not steadily or gracefully, in
the wheelchair, I felt as if I had crossed a minefield without detonating an
explosive.

By this time it was the end of January, too late for me to return to
school that semester, even if I recovered in the next few weeks. I had realized in the hospital that it would be impossible for me to attend classes that
spring and had accepted it. I believed the leave would be only temporary.
Throughout that winter and spring, I looked forward to going back to
school in the fall, and resuming the life I knew would be waiting for me.

When my parents and I pulled up to the house, they took the rented
wheelchair from the trunk. With great effort from me and help from my
father, I was transferred from the car to the wheelchair and brought inside.
Since I could not climb the steps to my bedroom, my parents had rented
a hospital bed, which they had placed in the living room. My grandmother
had donated my great-grandmother's walker, which I used inside the house
for the limited amount of walking of which I was capable. We installed a
built-up toilet seat in the bathroom on the first floor. Whenever I needed
to get out of bed, out of a chair, or even off the toilet seat, someone had to
assist me. My mother even cut up my food because my hands were too
weak to do it.

For the first day or two, my mom gave me sponge baths and washed
my hair in the sink. Then she suggested that she could wash my hair and
bathe me more thoroughly in the shower. We had a full bathroom with
a shower, including a built in shower seat, on the first floor, but I would
have to go down one small step into the indoor pool room, walk across the
room, then go up another small step into the bathroom. My parents, and
my grandparents, who were visiting at the time, assured me they would
hold me up as I used the walker to navigate the two steps. But as much as
I wanted that shower, I panicked at the thought of attempting the steps. I
was terrified of falling. Dr. Kostos's legacy to me. Until he left me on the
floor, I had not feared falling because I had never hurt myself, and someone
had always helped me to my feet. I was never blamed for the failure of my
limbs. After much crying on my part and encouragement on my parents', I
did reach the shower. But the experience was traumatic for us all.

After a few more days went by, I telephoned Dr. Kostos. My condition
was not improving, and my family and I were concerned. Though he had
treated me abominably in the hospital, Dr. Kostos was still the only physi-

cian who had my complete lupus history; it seemed to me that I had no other medical professional to whom I could turn. I felt trapped. But my call was also placed partly in hope. My fury about Dr. Kostos's actions that final night were mixed with memories of how Dr. Kostos had been so unfailingly kind, warm, and supportive for the past year and a half. I thought that perhaps I might again find the gentle doctor upon whose knowledge and compassion I had depended.

So I dialed the familiar number with mixed emotions: anticipation, apprehension, anger, and hurt. When I told Dr. Kostos that I was in no better shape than when I left the hospital, he informed me that my problems resulted from a stress reaction, not from any physical cause. I was probably traumatized because I had to leave school. I was also deconditioned, and he suggested that I begin my swimming regimen again. He did not advise me to seek the help of a psychiatrist. Implicitly, he was making himself quite clear that he considered these symptoms my responsibility. If I would just take hold of myself by accepting not being in school and by building my body back up through swimming, I would recover.

After he finished speaking, there was a moment of silence, and the small hope that I had harbored at the beginning of the conversation flickered and died. As I replaced the receiver, I felt as if I had fallen to the bottom of a deep, empty well. I tried to climb back to the surface, but could find no foothold. Trapped in the dark, I screamed for help. Someone arrived; I recognized and trusted him. I thought, "He will bring me to safety." He stood at the edge of the well and shone a blinding torch full upon my face. In its cold, white glare, he said, "You got yourself into the well. Get yourself out." Then he disappeared, leaving me helpless and alone.

The night following my conversation with Dr. Kostos, I spiked a fever of 103°. With no one else to consult, my parents contacted the urologist who had treated me the previous spring. He recommended a rheumatologist with whom he frequently worked. The urologist called his colleague, and I was given an appointment that day.

As I was wheeled into the waiting room, I was immediately struck by the furnishings, all expensive and tasteful Victorian reproductions. The room's two oversized leather armchairs, leather couch, cherry wood tables, and hunting scenes painted in dark oils lent the room the air of a gentleman's study. The nurse beckoned us to follow her to the doctor's office. Dr. John C. Warner, who appeared to be in his early sixties, was seated at his desk, his bearing ramrod straight. I was not surprised to learn that he had recently gone into private practice after spending most of his career at a prominent military hospital. During our conversation that afternoon and in the days that followed, he directed most of his comments to my family, especially to my father and my grandfather. I received the distinct impression that women, young ladies especially, but also older women, were meant to be seen but not heard. Though I did not exactly bond with Dr. Warner, he was at least willing to take my problems seriously. He wanted to hospitalize me immediately to discover the cause of my high fever and to find out what lay behind my severe weakness and diminished sensation.

The fever resolved almost as soon as I was admitted to the hospital, so Dr. Warner focused upon finding the cause of my severe weakness, diminished sensation, and continuing back pain. He called in a neurologist who performed an electromyogram (EMG), a test that measures the electrical activity of muscles and is used to diagnose neuromuscular disorders. The neurologist discovered evidence of an L4 ridiculopathy, which was indicative of some sort of spinal cord involvement. But no definitive diagnosis was made; no exact label for my symptoms was given.

Dr. Warner told my family and me that, whatever the root cause of my disability, we could not allow it to continue. We would place the issue of diagnosis on hold while we aggressively treated the disability by intensive rehabilitation. I began physical, occupational, and eventually aquatic therapy at a local rehabilitation center with which Dr. Warner was associated.

But before I visited the rehab center for the first time, my mother and my grandmother suggested a different form of therapy. My mother asked, "Would you like us to take you to the mall? We could use the wheelchair. It would be fun for you to get out." I leaped at her offer to take me shopping. I was tired of being inside hospitals, doctors' offices, or the house. I imagined myself fully recovered, wearing my new clothes to go out with my friends. I was too weak to try on the clothes in the stores, so my mother and grandmother just wheeled me around, and I picked out what I wanted. I got so excited that I nearly fell out of the wheelchair while reaching for an outfit I especially liked. My grandmother yanked me back by the collar just in time and yelled at me not to do that to her again. But her scolding was good natured. Both she and my mom were happy to see me taking so much pleasure in our outing.

Then I began the rehab program. My parents brought me in the morning, and I stayed most of the day. The schedule was as rigorous as I could tolerate. With alacrity and enthusiasm, I worked with the various therapists—mostly young women in their mid-twenties. I had always responded well to physical therapy, because it was an active form of intervention. Exercising was a chance for me to take positive control over my illness in several ways. The therapists taught me many practical techniques I could use to compensate for my deficits, so I could enjoy a higher level of functioning while my body healed. Through the process of strengthening muscles, regaining coordination, and improving balance, they were also instructing me about my body and how my nerves, joints, and muscles joined together to produce all the ordinary movements I had always taken for granted but now could no longer do. Knowledge was another way for me to regain some sense of control over my body.

I still can vividly recall my physical therapist, Debbie. She was barely five feet tall, but there was no question of her physical strength or authority. I used to call her, fondly (or not so fondly, depending on my mood) "Little Hitler"—behind her back, of course. She was tough and demanding, but she never asked for more than my body or I could give. And she cared. We kept in touch for a few years after my discharge, until my parents moved from Maryland.

It was she who cured me of my fear of falling. When she heard from my mother that I was terrified about falling, she firmly told me the next visit, "Melissa, your mom says you're afraid of falling. Well, with your balance and strength problems, it's bound to happen. I'm going to teach you ways to stop yourself from going down. If you do, then you need to know how to do it without hurting yourself. And you have to know how to get up with and without help. What if you're alone in the room? Now let's get to work." Knowing there was little point in arguing with her, I followed her instructions to tumble from the elevated mat to the one on the floor. By the end of a few sessions, I had regained my confidence and felt secure that if I fell, I could successfully drag myself to a stable chair or couch and use her methods to pull myself up.

Physical therapy was defined by such landmarks and successes—the session when I finally lost my fear of falling, progressing from the walker and wheelchair to two Canadian crutches (also called polio crutches, with their metal arm bands and handles for the fingers to grasp), then one crutch, a quad cane, and, finally, freedom from any adaptive equipment. Perhaps the most important gain for me was being able to drive a car again. My parents lived in a suburban, almost rural area. There was no public transportation. Driving was not a luxury but a necessity. Regaining my ability to drive was part of reestablishing my independence. But my progress, though steady, was slow. From the beginning, Dr. Warner was perplexed about the cause of my disability, and the pace of my recovery further baffled and troubled him.

At the beginning of April, when I was still using two Canadian crutches, Dr. Warner informed me, during one of the few appointments for which my parents did not stay with me during the meeting, that I was suffering from a conversion reaction. Though he believed that I had lupus, it was a stress response, not neurologic or any other involvement of my disease, that had caused my inability to walk, the severity of my weakness in my hands and arms, my problems with coordination, and my diminished sensation.

Dr. Warner invoked battle terminology to account for my hysteria. "I've seen a wide range of stress reactions from boys who come back from the front. The mind can powerfully affect the body." In his view, my own reaction stemmed from the stress of being in school. When I tried to communicate to him how much I delighted in my school life, he held up the silencing hand of a patriarch who is listening to an unruly child talking out of turn. "I remember a college student who wanted to go to medical school and asked me for a recommendation. He didn't get into medical school and committed suicide. Lot of pressure at school."

I did not argue any further with him; I could see that his mind was set. My parents picked me up at his office. As they drove me home, in some ways, I felt as if I had been transported back to the summer before I was diagnosed with lupus. The issues were the same, though the stakes were higher this time. The disability had been extreme. I had never been so ill or so physically helpless in my life. As in that summer before the diagnosis of lupus, the idea of mental illness as the cause of my physical problems was devastating to me. I was consumed by guilt and shame to think that I might have put myself and my family through such an ordeal because of some emotional lapse. I also knew, now, that physicians sometimes blamed the victim when the disease process could not be neatly identified or labeled. I felt angry to think that I might be the object of such blame again. I thought furiously, "I need to be concentrating on healing and not fighting my doctors."

When my family and I returned home, I told them what Dr. Warner had said. Their reaction mirrored my own. They were confused, angry, indignant, and frightened. But after we had calmed down, we all agreed that this was too important to dismiss. If I were suffering from an emotional reaction, it was essential to discover why I was troubled and find help for me. We assumed that an emotional problem, if left untreated, might cripple me again. None of us could bear the thought of that. My parents reassured me that no matter what happened and what we found, they loved me, did not blame me for the events of the past few months, and would always be there for me.

So, as in the months before I was diagnosed, I began the rounds of doctors, collecting and assembling information in order to make sense of the symptoms. I went to an orthopedist. Then I consulted another neurologist. Though he conducted several tests that revealed abnormalities in nerve conduction along my optic nerve and in several places along my spinal column, he too attributed my disability mainly, though not completely, to stress. According to him, this stress resulted from sexual frustration as well as my being unmarried and childless.

Next I went to see Evelyn McFadden again. Because she had come to know me the previous summer, I felt that she would have a good basis from which to judge my current mental state. I told her what my physicians had said and that I wanted her to give me a full mental evaluation. I had to know whether or not, in her opinion, I had some kind of mental block that needed to be addressed. She did as I asked, and after meeting with me for several weeks, she stated emphatically that she could see no signs of a conversion hysteria. She would write a report to Dr. Warner and asked for my permission to speak with him on the phone. To her surprise, when she contacted Dr. Warner, he was incredibly rude and condescending, refusing to give credence to anything she had to say.

I also consulted with my endocrinologist. Dr. Joshua has medical degrees in psychiatry and endocrinology as well as doctorates in biochemistry and immunology. I related Dr. Warner's and Dr. Kostos's conclusions and how they had reached them. Dr. Joshua rejected the idea of a conversion hysteria. "You're not suffering from a conversion hysteria. If you want to see a psychiatrist for an evaluation, I can refer you to several excellent ones. But you would be treating Dr. Kostos's and Dr. Warner's problem, not your own!"

Dr. Joshua said that he could explain the disability resulting from this past flare, at least in general terms. He said that, furthermore, if an emotional block were present, it would be highly unlikely for me to make any significant improvement physically, because we would not be treating the true underlying problem. "Is stress affecting your physical state?" asked Dr. Joshua. "Absolutely. Is it contributing in some way to your illness? Sure. Did stress cause your inability to walk, or your diminishing of sensation? No."

Dr. Joshua's partner, who also rendered his opinion, pointed out the corresponding gains in therapy with improvements in thyroid tests and sedimentation rates. He believed both thyroid and neurological involvement lay behind my symptoms and disability of the past few months.

Finally I discussed my situation with my physical therapists. They had worked with me every day for several months, and I felt that they knew me and my body. I had developed a profound respect for their expertise. All agreed without question that there were serious neurological problems.

At this point my family and I decided that the diagnosis of conversion hysteria made no sense, and we stopped our investigations. I was furious with Warner for planting such tearing self-doubts in my mind and sending me and my family on such an emotionally, physically, and financially draining goose chase. But I could not change rheumatologists; I needed him in order to stay enrolled in the rehab program that was putting me back on my feet. So I tolerated Warner, seeing as little of him as possible. On June 12 I beat Debbie in a game of tennis. Her loss was a triumph for us both. I was discharged that day.

Three days later I dismissed Dr. Warner in a meeting that I am sure he has not forgotten. Though I never raised my voice, used any foul language, or lowered myself to accusations of any kind, I had the ultimate temerity to challenge his authority. In a calm, analytical way, I laid out my evidence, which contradicted his conversion hysteria theory. Instead of responding in kind and discussing the points I had made, he turned a rather interesting shade of purple and said, "You're the one who is disturbed, so you can't make any judgments on your own state of mind. These other people aren't rheumatologists, so they can't tell me how to make my diagnosis. And if you want to surround yourself with a bunch of people who feed your delusional fantasies, then go right ahead!" I only said coolly, refusing to get rattled, "Well, I can see there is nothing more to discuss." With my head held high and my bearing as straight and proud as his own, I left his office.

Of course, when I got into my car, it was a full fifteen minutes before I stopped shaking and felt fit to drive. But as I drove the familiar route from his office to my parents' house, I realized that the nightmare was finally behind me. I opened my window and breathed deeply of the early summer air, cleansing my being of the months past. I pressed my foot on the accelerator, joyfully feeling the car propelling me forward, forward.

11
Oasis

Summer 1990

My slumbering senses awaken from dark wintry sleep
when icy illness blanketed all in silencing snow.
Like one of spring's flowers I open out to sun
reveling in exquisite sensations,
breezes brushing delicately over my face,
carpet rough against my bared feet,
kittens' fur such softness to my hungry fingertips,
a new dimension to my world.

My drowsy limbs come out of their cold sleep
while nerves and muscles made mute regain their voice,
singing with wonder at winter's abatement.
I grasp a spoon, rise from a chair, climb a step,
best of all feel my legs carry me with certainty and strength;
each time I am reborn in joy.

Yet even as the grip of winter eases,
I think about the turning of the seasons
and wonder when winter will come again.
But I will not chill spring and summer hours
with thoughts of returning autumn.
When winter days come cold and dreary,
I will warm myself
with thoughts of spring.

THE SUMMER of 1990 was a time of being and beginnings. I savored every aspect of my physical recovery. I also began my independent study with Dr. Stein, or Esther, as she had asked me to call her. We had telephoned each another and kept up such correspondence as I was able during the winter and spring, planning that I would start an independent study course with her in earnest during the summer.

Over those frightening, dreary, and frustrating months of flare and recovery, my friendship with Esther had grown considerably. She offered her compassion and support partly because it was in her nature to do so. But our relationship and the work we did together over the years also stemmed from some similarities in our personal histories and interests. Like me, Esther came from a loving Jewish family. When she was seventeen, she was stricken by polio and was gravely ill. She recovered, but walked with a limp. She knew about serious, long-term illness and disability from her own experience. Like mine, her parents became protective after her illness, thinking of Esther as their wounded child. She, too, needed to reconcile her parents to her need for independence as she grew into young adulthood.

As I described earlier, Esther was a genuine scholar, with interests spanning the arts and sciences. She had a true passion for literature and had studied it extensively in college. My own love for literature lived as an abiding faith in me. At the university, I immersed myself in the literature created by different nations, eras, and writers. As I continued to hone my literary skills and expand my background, I realized that I primarily wanted to study literature by placing it in a large framework, mainly as part of the history of ideas. I wished to examine the relationship between literature and the society from which it comes. Even more fundamentally, I wished to explore the vital connection between literature and the human condition, a bond transcending time and culture.

Because of my personal experiences, I was becoming increasingly interested in the medical world. This interest merged with my longtime love for literature and my conviction that I wanted ultimately to view literature with a wide lens. In Esther I found a true mentor. We decided that we would spend the summer reading works with medical themes. She would provide her extensive sociological training—including her specialty in medical sociology—her literary acumen, and her enthusiasm, and I could bring my literary knowledge to our discussions that we conducted over the phone and through the mail.

We began by reading a sociology of medicine text written by Esther. She wanted to give me a grounding in some of the field's fundamental research. Her book is divided into seven chapters: "The Social and Cultural Significance of Health and Illness," "The Professions of Medicine and Nursing," "The Education, Training, and Socialization of Physicians: Medical School," "The Education, Training, and Socialization of Physicians: Residency and Practice," "The Hospital: A Social and Cultural Microcosm," "Medical Science and Medical Research," and "The Sociology of Bioethics." She also sent me articles written by other sociologists. In this way, for the first few weeks of my independent study we used sociology as a base for investigating the various topics and themes we would later encounter and examine in literary works.

Throughout the summer we continued to read sociological works and articles, but we added into our studies diverse works of literature in some way related to the subjects of health, illness, and medicine. We began with a classic novel that has great relevance in the age of AIDS: *The Plague,* by Albert Camus, in which unfolds the story of a town's battle with bubonic plague. Then we moved on to Thomas Mann's *The Magic Mountain,* which depicts life at a tuberculosis sanatorium. Alexander Solzhenitzyn's *Cancer Ward* was the next novel on our list. We also found an entire category of works, some more literary than others, written by physician authors such as Walker Percy, William Carlos Williams, Perri Klass, Richard Selzer, Oliver Sacks, and Samuel Shem. Their writings include novels, poetry, short stories, literary nonfiction, and works not easily categorized.

We approached these texts by combining as full a literary analysis as we were able with our interest in understanding the work in light of the medical themes with which it dealt. We both strongly felt that we could be satisfied only by this dual perspective. For example, Thomas Mann captures the realities of a tuberculosis sanatorium with as much technical accuracy as a sociologist. Like a social scientist, he gathered data for his work by performing a kind of participant observation; he based his novel on observations made while visiting his wife at a tuberculosis sanatorium. Yet *The Magic Mountain* is not a sociological text. It is a great work of literary art and must be treated as such.

But what are the elements that differentiate Mann's work from an extremely well-written ethnographic account of life in a tuberculosis sanatorium before World War I? This question is not so easily answered. A social scientist might have taken the same set of materials—participant observation, research, insights, and analysis in order to produce a powerfully, perhaps even lyrically written ethnography that would contribute to our knowledge of the subject. It might be equally valuable in its own way, but it would not be art. Why not?

Curiosity about the artistic process became an integral part of our reading. It came to the fore when we studied William Carlos Williams, a favorite writer of mine. Williams directly uses his experiences as a practicing physician to create poetry, short stories, and other writings. But his works are neither transcriptions nor analytical treatments by a sociologist. His manner of transforming his daily life into art fascinated me.

That summer I reveled in the oasis created by my physical recovery, my studies, and my growing friendship with Esther. But after my initial happiness at finding myself in this place, I felt troubled by anger, hurt, and pain—reactions to my experiences that winter, especially to the way in which I had recently been treated by various health professionals, mainly Dr. Kostos and Dr. Warner. There were other feelings, too, some I couldn't even identify. All were emotions I had not fully faced or even acknowledged during those months of flare and recovery when I had been reserving my energies to fight the physical disease.

I knew it was now time to face what had happened. At first I did so on an intellectual level. I began by using my powers of analysis in an attempt to comprehend my physicians' actions. The past lay behind me in a confusing, tangled jumble in which I had often played the role of helpless victim. The past was immutable, but I hoped that my gaining further insight might prevent me from getting caught up in similar situations in the future. In this way, the acquisition of knowledge could give me some feeling of being in charge of my life again. I thought that such empowerment would help dispel the anger in me, a fury fueled by the feelings of powerlessness and impotence inspired by Drs. Kostos and Warner in particular.

As I struggled to discern how and why the events of the past winter and spring had taken place, I found no easy answers. There was only a complicated interweaving of possible causes and motivations that included and went beyond the individual personality traits, biases, and skills of the physicians involved. First I focused on Dr. Kostos, because my anger, fed by a deep hurt, was directed more strongly toward him than toward Dr. Warner. When I thought of my hospital stay with Dr. Kostos, I knew that he had exercised poor medical judgment by failing to investigate the cause of my falling, diminished sensation, and pronounced weakness. All those symptoms were glibly assumed to be the result of deconditioning. And the bladder symptoms, which, in conjunction with back pain and loss of sensation from toes to waist, can be classic signs of problems with the spinal cord, were never thought to be anything but the product of an infection. Simple diagnostic error did not fully explain Dr. Kostos's assessment of my condition; he seemed to be incapable of even considering that my disease might be taking on a new form. Why?

After thinking about our doctor-patient relationship, I decided that part of the problem stemmed from his caring too much—an ironic conclusion, when I thought of how much pain he had inflicted on me. Clearly he identified me with his daughter, who was almost exactly my age. He often spoke to me about her, emphasizing our similarities. She was ambitious and very involved in school; she worked hard. When I spoke of my concerns about staying in school and having enough energy to enjoy a rich, productive life there, he would say, "Oh, you are just like my daughter, always worrying."

I believe that Dr. Kostos's seeing me as a young woman much like his beloved daughter proved to be disastrous. He became too emotionally involved to maintain the objectivity he needed to accurately diagnose and treat. Dr. Kostos was also working under the tremendous pressure of trying to control an acute phase of lupus, a disease whose course is extremely erratic and uncertain and whose treatment is highly variable. Both his loss of objectivity and the inherent nature of the disease caused Dr. Kostos's reaction. Instead of dealing with my medical problems in an appropriate fashion, he withdrew himself emotionally, then blamed me for my illness.

At least Dr. Warner took my symptoms and my disability seriously. He made a real attempt to diagnose my weakness, diminished sensation, and back pain by taking x-rays and calling upon neurologists in the hospital, and he did prescribe the intensive rehabilitation, without which I firmly believe I would not have recovered the use of my limbs. But ultimately, Dr. Warner also blamed me for my disability.

His response was not unlike Dr. Smith's. Dr. Warner could not label my symptoms with the military precision his medical training, and personality, I suspect, demanded. Frustrated, he burdened me with the responsibility for all that had taken place and so absolved himself from what he would have perceived as an uncomfortable failure to neatly explain, clarify, and document down to the last detail—an underlying expectation of the modern medical professional.

Not only had both physicians blamed me for my illness; they had also used my age as a way to do so. Each physician had recounted horror stories of young adults who had succumbed to the stresses of university life and died. Dr. Kostos had told me about his young patient who, not wanting to have a "moon face" (the common rounding of the face due to steroids) now that she was in college, had stopped her prednisone suddenly. Dr. Warner had described the young man who had committed suicide while pursuing plans for medical school. The physicians had depicted in graphic detail the pressures of school, but they did not ask me how *I* felt about school and life—*me, Melissa,* an individual, not a representative of a particular age group. In their minds, they reduced me to a type, a cardboard figure with predictable responses, who could be found at fault and dismissed.

The neurologist who had asked about my sex life had done much the same thing. Although his tests had revealed demyelinization of the nerves in the spinal cord and the optic nerve, he still searched for explanations of my condition in my status as a young adult female who might be prone, because of her age and sex, to outbursts of hysteria. In other unpleasant encounters, I found that physicians were uncomfortable with my age or sex (or both) and made certain quick assumptions about my identity based on these factors. Over the spring, I visited a Ph.D.-trained psychologist to receive instruction in hypnosis and biofeedback for pain control and for my Raynaud's. I responded very well to the techniques. After I had mastered them, the psychologist suggested that I might lose five pounds in order to be more attractive to men. Then I would date more often, have a more active sex life, and my lupus symptoms would disappear!

As I thought about the events of the winter and spring, at last I felt I had come to some important understandings. I realized that lupus, with all its high degree of uncertainty, its elusive character, places a great burden upon physicians who sometimes react by turning on the patient. In my case, they did this by placing me in the pigeonhole "young adult female." We have neonatal, pediatric, adolescent, adult, and geriatric medicine. But young adulthood, although rarely recognized as a separate branch of medicine, presents its own special issues and challenges for patients and physicians alike.

My insights led me to make some decisions concerning my future. I realized that I must insist on my health-care professionals' treating me as Melissa—not as a copy of someone else and not according to their ideas about a "typical" young adult female. I would not allow myself to be forced into some prefabricated category. I also wanted to let my physicians know my own expectations at the outset of our relationship. I did not expect them to be perfect, omniscient, or able to provide immediate explanations and solutions to all my physical problems. I could accept the unknown if they could. But I did demand their best skill and that they approach me with patience and, most of all, with respect. In coming to these conclusions, I had a better sense of order and control. I felt some of my anger leave me.

But I needed to deal with the events of the winter and spring on an emotional as well as an intellectual level. Once again I turned to Evelyn McFadden for help. The kindness in her voice, her relaxed body language, the gentle touch of her hands on mine, her soft blue gaze that invited me to confide in her—all contributed to create a conduit that allowed my pain, hurt, sense of outrage, and grief to flow from me in words, tears, and even in humor. She offered me empathetic guidance. But toward the end of the summer, I decided that I needed to talk to one more person before I could fully come to terms, if that were at all possible, with my experiences. I wrote to Dr. Kostos.

I did not do so out of petty spite, and I did not expect a reply. But I wanted to hold him accountable for his actions. I wanted him to know how much he had hurt me, even if he had not intended it, and how mistaken he had been in his diagnosis. I asked that he would not stereotype his young adult patients and that he would think seriously before putting another young person through the same ordeal. I told him that I had recovered and was eager to return to school and all the excitement school life held for me. I just hoped that if I ever became so ill again, that this time there would be a competent and compassionate physician working with me. He never answered my letter.

I wish I could say that by the close of summer, I completely forgave, forgot, and moved blithely onward, unmarked by the events of the past months. But life only works that way in a bad TV movie of the week. I did succeed in letting go much of my pain and anger. Yet even though my fury had been dispelled, my distrust of physicians remained. I never again wanted to make myself vulnerable to another physician.

Dear Doctor,
I came to your office today.

My body was broken, sore
so I brought it to
you.

With me, came my spirit.
I tried to leave it home,
for it is healthy,
joyous.

I did not want
to expose its softness
to the doctor's often
sharp tongue
which can form
piercing words
that cut more thoroughly
than any scalpel made.
An incision left from this
slash
is so slow to heal,
its stitches tearing
under the least pressure,
exposing the hideous
wound.
Many tongue lashings
have I received from you
gentle healers;
my spirit is criss-crossed with
knotty scars.

Each time a doctor strikes me,
I think the pain
will be less
from familiarity.
Yet each time the
gash
yields blood.

My spirit tissue,
strong, resilient,
filled with life,
has healed from
the most brutal attacks.
Yet how many times
can my spirit regenerate?

So I tried to come
to you body only,
keeping my tender spirit
from harm.
But it would not keep away.
So I beg you,
do not
rip at my soul.
It has endured
enough.

Perhaps your spirit
can reach out for mine,
finding what is familiar,
another human soul.
So let us meet
in peace.

So let us meet / in peace. A wish that has not always been granted. Certainly not by Dr. Fields and Dr. Gresley. Yet as I write these lines, collecting and sifting through the scattered pieces of memory, insight, and reflection, I feel my anger lessen. Though I cannot tell the final shape these recollections will take, I believe they will create a coherent whole that will bring me understanding. And peace. I am following the river, coming ever closer to its source, secret of this desert land.

Through my discussions with Evelyn I came to understand that I did not fear only physicians: I also feared my future. Though I was sure that I had not suffered from a conversion hysteria, I did not know what had caused many of my symptoms that winter. I knew that I had experienced a severe lupus flare, but had the lupus inflamed my central nervous system? Could I have another such attack? Could I do anything to prevent a recurrence? Would the lupus involve other organ systems, causing even more gruesome problems? How far should I go in my efforts to answer these questions?

As the summer drew to a close, these fears and questions occupied my mind more frequently. Finally, one day while I was swimming, as the even, rhythmic strokes steadied my careening thoughts, words became images, remembered and new. Once again I found my way into my future.

In my imagination I walked freely through a color-drenched field, the place of this spring's recovery. I drifted among tender blooms still curled slightly toward the center, whose fresh fragrance was that of the early morning. The swaying, emerald grass felt soft against my legs and the earth deliciously damp and cool beneath my feet, between my toes. A field just after sunrise when all has begun again, and everything seems possible.

But "my beautiful field was ringed by deep woods / Where lurked unknown dangers and mysteries." Even as I reveled in my field, "I sensed an enemy's presence close by. / Fetid breath surrounded me. Though unseen / His devilish existence I couldn't deny." I gazed out at those forbidding woods, where the leaves grew black and curled on trees set close together, making a formidable barrier to sunlight and hope. I knew that there the wolf waited for me.

I looked in that bleak landscape for the flashing yellow eyes, the limbs lean and long. As I strained to see, searching the woods all around me, I gradually became aware how mesmerizing was the darkness and how easy it would be to lose myself there, ignoring all that my field had to offer. With an enormous effort, I wrenched my gaze from the woods and the wolf.

And in that turning away, I freed myself, at least for the moment. I reaffirmed my dedication to the Present, and in being able to do so, I was now ready to move forward. I eagerly made my preparations to return to school. Happy and anxious, my parents watched me fill my suitcases and shop for last-minute items as the days of August disappeared. There was no question, in their minds or mine, whether or not I should go back to the university, but that did not mean they were not fearful about what my future might hold in store for me. Their memories of the past months were just as vivid as mine.

During those months, they had cared for me as when I was a very small child. They had bathed and fed me, and pushed me in a chair as one does for a baby in a stroller. For a time, they had made many of the major medical decisions, because I had not the awareness or the strength to do so. But now I had regained my independence, and my parents needed to find the strength to let me use it. We celebrated my birthday before I left Maryland. As always, my parents were generous with their presents, but the greatest gift, given with much love and pain, was their letting me go when it was time.

When we arrived at my dormitory, the car finally unloaded, my mother held me in a tight embrace, as if she could not bear to release me. Then

I pull away.
In anguish she feels her empty arms fall to her side,
but then as she follows me with her gaze,
she sees her child grown,
realizing she has kept a mother's only promise,
the certainty of her love and the uncertainty of life.
I turn to her and smile;
we are joined together
healed.

12

Setting Forth Again

Fall 1990 – Spring 1991

I RETURNED to my life at the university. All was delightfully familiar—my friends, classes, parties, the dorm activities at Washington
House. Though I found this world to be much the same as it had been
when I left it those months ago, everything in it seemed filled with an added
sweetness. Each morning when I sauntered down Laurel Walk, with its
bower of trees and cobblestone path, a quiet but profound pleasure came
over me. With a smile on my lips, I would think, "I'm here. I'm back."

By now I accepted the fact that the university, for all its magic and
charm, could not shield me from the lupus. However much I disliked the
idea of seeking out yet another rheumatologist and spending more precious
time and energy on my illness, I knew that I had to have a physician to call
in case of an emergency. My symptoms were by no means gone; I was not
in remission. But the disease was at least much more stable than it had been.
I planned to find a rheumatologist, discuss my history, and then contact
him or her only if the need arose.

I collected names of rheumatologists in the city and scheduled appointments with three. After my recent experiences, I wanted to choose carefully
and wisely. At first I was hesitant to interview a rheumatologist at CGH, the
hospital so closely associated with Laurel University. I felt awkward about
receiving my care from a hospital located only a few blocks away from my
dorm. Previously, I had tried to maintain a strict division between my "illness life" and my "normal life." Physical distance, a geographical separation,
between the hospital where Dr. Kostos practiced and Laurel University had
made this easier to manage, emotionally and practically. At CGH, I feared

encountering friends or faculty members as I went into and came out of the hospital and being asked questions I might not want to answer. I would not enjoy the same privacy as before.

But Esther, who was associated with the university's medical school as well as its sociology department, asked if I would like her to speak with her friend, the dean of the medical school. The dean recommended a rheumatologist at CGH. Despite my reservations, I decided to give CGH a try.

It was the middle of September. My mom came in from Maryland for the day to meet the rheumatologist, Dr. Averapporti. Though not at all luxurious, the waiting room was clean and bright. The staff, consisting of the secretaries, the nurse, the residents, and the doctors, created a pleasant atmosphere. The secretaries and the nurse greeted patients with friendliness, often chatting with the ones they knew. Physicians walked their patients out to the front desk, answering last-minute questions or giving instructions in a relaxed, caring way.

Still, I waited with frozen hands and a hammering heart. Fifteen or twenty minutes after my arrival, a doctor emerged from the examining room area, accompanied by the patient with whom he had just had an appointment. The name tag on the doctor's jacket identified him as Dr. Averapporti. As he said good-bye to his patient, I watched and listened, trying to form an impression.

His physical appearance was striking. His long white coat accentuated his tall, slim frame and dark, chiseled Roman features. He looked young, perhaps in his late twenties, though his secretary had told me when I scheduled my visit that he was thirty-five. Perhaps what was most noticeable was his expression and manner. The patient, a middle-aged woman, was obviously distressed and discouraged about her illness. Dr. Averapporti's attitude was kind, sympathetic, and encouraging—not condescending or impatient. He reminded her of the plan they would follow. If it did not work, she should not hesitate to call him, and they would explore other options. While they talked, his hand rested on her shoulder.

After she left, he walked over to me and said with a warm smile and a handshake, "Melissa Goldstein? So sorry to have kept you waiting. Won't you come this way?" Then he led me off to an examining room. The room was relatively small and crowded. Bookshelves overflowing with medical texts, journals, and plastic models of joints lined the left-hand wall as one entered the room. In the middle of the room was a wooden desk piled with papers. Opposite the desk were two chairs like those in the waiting room. The examining table and a sink were located inconspicuously against the wall to the right of the door. The windows, which I faced as I entered the room, overlooked the university building where I had taken history classes. I felt as if I were in a professor's office rather than an examining room, and the almost academic setting was soothing to me.

Dr. Averapporti asked, "So, what brings you here today?" I pulled out a several-page medical history that I had written, copies of test results, and a short list of questions. As quickly and concisely as I could, I told my medical story, using my written copy for backup. I explained that I was doing relatively well at present; I just needed someone to consult if there were any problems in the future. Dr. Averapporti sometimes stopped me for clarification of specific points, but mostly he listened with a complete, empathetic attention that invited me to confide in him.

After I had finished, he said that he would step out of the room for a few minutes so that I could change into a gown. While Dr. Averapporti and I had been talking, I had become less tense, but as I shed my clothes and donned the gown, my wariness and fears returned. I felt very uneasy about being examined by a physician. As I looked out the window at the college campus, I wished I were outside on my way to class. Anywhere but in this office.

Dr. Averapporti returned. He examined me thoroughly, but his touch was very gentle. As he looked at my rashes, manipulated my joints, and tested my muscles and reflexes, he kept up an easy, steady stream of conversation. We spoke about my life at school, my family, my growing up in Maryland. He explained that he had just begun work at CGH and was originally from New York. Gradually, I felt more relaxed. When he was finished, he told me that I could get dressed while he brought my mother back from the waiting room.

My mother and Dr. Averapporti soon arrived, and Dr. Averapporti gave us his opinion. "I definitely agree with the diagnosis of lupus. However, I'm concerned about the symptoms you're still experiencing, especially in light of your history. I realize that everything becomes relative, and compared to what you've been through, your current problems don't seem that significant to you. But I think that these symptoms need to be dealt with. Your gastric symptoms especially worry me, because they were so severe in the past. I'd like to begin by getting complete blood studies. Then I'd like to send you to a gastroenterologist here at CGH. Your stomach problems could be the result of the lupus or an unrelated illness. Just because you have lupus, it doesn't mean that you can't have other illnesses. It's important that we rule out any other disorders, so we'll know how to treat you."

Though I did not relish the idea of visiting more doctors and spending more time in the world of illness, his approach and reasoning did make sense to me. He had treated me with respect and consideration during our meeting. Instinctively, I felt that Dr. Averapporti was a person I could come to trust. I thought we would be able to work together.

But before I made my final decision, I had a few questions and comments. First, I wanted to know if he relied solely, or predominantly, on blood work to define lupus activity. I explained that my blood counts had never been reliable indicators of lupus activity. He responded by saying that each patient was different in his or her presentation, and that he would gauge the lupus activity and make treatment decisions based on my reporting of symptoms and his clinical examination combined with blood work or other tests that might be needed. That seemed reasonable to me.

Then, taking a deep breath, I gave him my final test. I looked him straight in the eye and said, "Dr. Averapporti, I just want you to know that I don't expect you to be omniscient or have perfect solutions or even absolute explanations at hand for every one of my symptoms. My case has been complicated, and it hasn't always been clear what's been going on. I do understand the difficulties involved in treating this disease. What I expect are your best efforts and your patience. I also always want you to be honest with me." I waited to see how he would react. He was not offended. He held my gaze, smiled, and replied, "That sounds fair enough." I thought to myself, "I've found a rheumatologist."

Mom agreed with my decision. Later that day, I canceled the other two rheumatology appointments and scheduled a follow-up visit with Dr. Averapporti for the next month. His office also made an appointment for me with the gastroenterologist. She was the first of several specialists to whom Dr. Averapporti referred me that fall and winter, for all my symptoms, which had abated, though never disappeared during the late spring and summer, slowly returned with gathering force. Dr. Averapporti sent me to his colleagues, using their specific knowledge to gather more information to guide him in treating me. One question that continually needed to be asked was whether or not a particular problem was lupus related. Because lupus can mimic many other diseases, we could not presume that it was always the culprit. Also, at this stage of our relationship, Dr. Averapporti was getting to know me, my body, and my disease. He was trying to learn the pattern of my illness, and he enlisted the help of his colleagues to do so.

Though I was sent to an ophthalmologist, a dermatologist, a neurologist, a pulmonary specialist, an endocrinologist, and a gynecologist all within the first six months of my initial meeting with Dr. Averapporti, I never felt that my care was fragmented. Dr. Averapporti coordinated all of the doctors' efforts, pulling the pieces of the diagnostic puzzle together and organizing my overall treatment plan.

By November my regimen included a dose of prednisone every other day. Dr. Averapporti decided to administer the drug every other day in order to minimize the steroid's side effects. When prednisone is taken on alternate days, the body still has to manufacture its own cortisone, the adrenal glands do not shut down, and the body does not become completely dependent on prednisone. The dosage was relatively small, but I felt ambivalent about taking the drug at all. It did provide some relief, however, and I hoped it would prevent the lupus from raging out of control.

On the other hand, I was only too aware of all the potential side effects, both short- and long-term. Within a year of taking steroids, I developed osteoporosis in my feet. I struggled with weight gain and fluid retention, spending as much time as I could exercising, mainly swimming and taking long walks. Each morning I would look in the mirror, anxiously searching for signs of the notorious "moon face." Another common side effect of steroids is mood changes. I rode waves of euphoria and crashed against rocks of irritability and weepiness. So my relationship with steroids was, and has remained, one of love and hate—love for the relief the steroids can bring and hate for the price they exact for their service.

During that fall and spring semester of 1990–1991, Dr. Averapporti and I were slowly forging our doctor-patient relationship. It was a time of learning for us both. He was gaining knowledge about my disease, how it manifested itself in my body and how it responded to various treatments. He was also getting to know me, the individual apart from her illness. In turn I was getting a sense of him and his personality, as well as his approach to diagnosis and treatment.

But in any relationship, there are issues to be worked through, and that was certainly the case between Dr. Averapporti and me. I did not communicate freely with him. Much to his frustration, I would not call immediately when my symptoms became worse; when I did finally call or arrive at the office for a visit, I minimized my problems. I had come to Dr. Averapporti heavily burdened by my past negative experiences. My respect for and trust in him grew as the months passed, but, still, part of me was always kept in watchful reserve. This part of me wondered if I could really depend on Dr. Averapporti, even though he seemed to be such a kind, intelligent physician. So I refrained from calling him when I should have, preferring to keep my disease to myself rather than risk hurt or betrayal.

However, my hesitancy about calling involved more than my fears of rejection or blame. I had returned to school and was committed to leading as full and satisfying a life there as I possibly could. I did not want illness to dominate my existence. I did not want to become the kind of patient who called in a panic every time her toe gave a twitch. Of course, I did not want to ignore the disease and let it flare out of control, either. But deciding when to call the doctor, and when to just manage on my own was a constant and difficult dilemma. To complicate matters further, many of my symptoms came and went; after a few days, they would disappear. I did not want to call the doctor or medicate for those manifestations of the disease. Also, my symptoms typically worsened, sometimes dramatically, during the pre-menstrual part of my cycle and usually improved once my period arrived. So each month I resisted calling the doctor, trying to hold on until my hormones provided some relief.

But many times when I waited, the symptoms became progressively worse, not better. By the time I contacted Dr. Averapporti, they were quite severe. When Dr. Averapporti would ask me when the symptoms first started, he would become quite upset that I had not called him much earlier. When the symptoms were still mild, though, I had no way of knowing whether they would simply fade away or quickly take me into a tailspin. I tried to keep a delicate balance between listening to my body's warnings signals with tuning my body out so that I could go about my daily round. That balance was never easy to maintain, and I always tended to err on the side of drowning out my body's danger calls in order to go forward with my life.

Reporting on my symptoms in the doctor's office was as problematic as deciding whether or not to make a telephone call to Dr. Averapporti. Usually I visited Dr. Averapporti every month. Between appointments, I would experience many different symptoms. The time we could spend together was limited, especially after the hospital put pressure on the rheumatology department to see a greater number of patients each day to bring in more money. Theoretically, Dr. Averapporti should have spent only ten to fifteen minutes on a routine appointment with an established patient, but his specialty was lupus. Since he mainly treated people with complicated, chronic illnesses, ten to fifteen minutes was an impossibly short allotment. He was a conscientious, dedicated physician who wanted to give his patients the attention they needed, so he gave more time to each person than the system allowed. He was continually running late.

Even though he gave extra time, with my array of symptoms, I had to carefully prioritize what we were going to talk about. If, for example, I decided that the gastric symptoms were my main problem at the moment, I would gloss over the rest of the symptoms, saving them for another visit. I would leave, and sometimes symptoms I had mentioned only in passing, or not discussed at all, went quickly from being on a low simmer to boiling over. If I then called Dr. Averapporti, he would exclaim, "I just saw you! Why didn't you talk about this when you were in my office?"

Dr. Averapporti spoke to me about his concerns that I was not calling him when I should and that I was denying the seriousness of my disease. He was worried that my behavior was interfering with my care. His nurse even pulled me aside after one appointment, telling me Dr. Averapporti was very distressed that I was not being open enough with him. I felt awful when I heard that, and at my next appointment I tried to explain why I delayed calling. I assured him that it was not because I did not trust *him*, but because I had been hurt in the past by other physicians. I also did not want to be consumed by my disease. I wanted to be as independent as possible; I did not want to call in if it was not absolutely necessary. I realized that I needed to do a better job about keeping him informed, and I would work on that.

I decided that the best way to open the channels of communication between Dr. Averapporti and me was through my old friend, poetry. At the end of my next appointment, I handed him three poems, "The Wolf," "My Garden," and "My Enemies." Dr. Averapporti said, "I don't know much about poems, but I'd be happy to read them." During the next visits, I waited for him to make some response. It became apparent that he had read the poems from his use of my metaphorical term "wolf" for the disease, yet he never made any explicit remarks.

Finally I asked him what he thought of my work. "I really enjoyed the poems" was his only comment. But later, I learned that he had circulated the poems around the office. From there, they made their way to various departments in the hospital. During office visits and hospital stays, physicians, nurses, and medical students tentatively approached me and asked if we could talk about my poems. The poems acted as pathways of communication, opening subjects and discussions which would normally have been taboo. We could share, in a safe, controlled way, our mutual frustrations, fears, and anger that the wolf refused to come under control.

In the spring of 1991 I was asked to speak to several classes of CGH medical students in their "Introduction to Clinical Medicine" course. I answered questions first from a panel of physicians, then from students, concluding with readings from my poems. The reception was overwhelmingly positive. The students felt that the poems, more than anything else that I had said, gave them insight into my experiences as a chronically ill young adult.

Over time my writing and my medical care became an integrated whole. Today throughout my medical chart, one finds my poems and even an essay. They are as much a part of my medical history as blood test results, x-ray reports, and physicians' notes. The biomedical data and my doctor's summaries document the physical changes wrought by the disease as well as the many medical regimens we have used, but my poems record, in my own voice, what those symptoms and treatments meant to me—the ways in which the illness altered how I thought of myself, my relationships to others, and my place in the world. At times, the poems have even guided Dr. Averapporti in making medical decisions by allowing him to understand how I truly felt about the illness as well as the various treatments, with their risks and benefits.

By allowing me to convey the experience of illness in a way that a description of the physical manifestation of disease could not capture, poetry opened up my relationships with my health-care professionals. Poetry had served me in a similar way with Dr. Kostos, but in my interactions with Dr. Averapporti and the other health-care professionals at CGH, poetry played an even more fundamental role in my medical care and my illness experiences.

What truly startled me, though, was my discovery that this medical community's response to poetry and writing was not passive. Numerous doctors, nurses, physical therapists, and other health-care professionals in the medical center were actively engaged in creative writing. Some were taking writing classes. They were eager to discuss literature with me, and a few asked if I would read their work.

During a hospital visit in the spring of 1991, I remember a rather enthusiastic medical student's pulling up a chair beside my hospital bed and speaking at great length about his love for the Brontë sisters' novels, particularly *Wuthering Heights*. Medical school afforded him little time to read and talk about literature, something he had always enjoyed, so he greatly appreciated this chance to chat. I, too, took great pleasure in the discussion, but I must admit, at that moment, I might have appreciated sleep even more!

While very flattering, these positive reactions to my work and my background in writing did not lead me to the conclusion that my poems would become classics or that I was destined to be a literary guru. Instead, the response of many members of this medical community alerted me to their attraction to literature, an interest which I had unwittingly tapped into through my own poetry. During my summer studies with Esther I had begun to explore the relationship between medicine and literature, and I continued my research with her throughout the 1990–1991 academic year. I found that my own experiences could be placed within the context of a rich, profound, and enduring relationship between medicine and the arts, especially literature.

I became especially interested in two examples of this relationship between medicine and the arts—the literary tradition of the physician as writer and the incorporation of the arts in *JAMA* (*Journal of the American Medical Association*). I found that the ranks of physician writers included such illustrious figures as François Rabelais, Tobias Smollett, John Keats, Gustave Flaubert, Anton Chekhov, Arthur Conan Doyle, Oliver Wendell Holmes, Somerset Maugham, and William Carlos Williams, to mention only a few. I studied their works, attempting to discover the diverse ways, both subtle and more obvious, in which their training and practice as physicians shaped their writings.

I also discovered that the link between medicine and the arts is not just a relic of the past; the relationship continues to thrive in *JAMA,* the most widely circulated medical journal in the world. The journal's primary purpose is to communicate and promote the science and practice of medicine. One would not expect the arts to be an integral and regular part of *JAMA,* yet on its cover, the journal displays fine art, of museum quality, usually a painting, sometimes a piece of sculpture. Accompanying the selected work of art is a full-page essay about the artist and his or her life, techniques, and themes.

The most powerful cover I have seen was actually a blank page. It appeared on the July 10, 1996, issue. Dr. Therese Southgate writes in her cover essay,

> Some things are seen best not in their presence, but in their absence. Thus, this issue of THE JOURNAL, which is dedicated to original research and other papers in HIV/AIDS, has as its cover not the usual reproduction of a work of fine art, but no art at all. *A Cover Without Art* is designed to highlight the toll the virus has taken among artists and other creative persons who have died prematurely because of AIDS. But there is another, incalculable cost as well—the loss to all those whose lives would have been

touched, even changed, but were not, by books not read because
they were never written, by paintings not seen because they were
never painted, by performances never heard because the song was
not sung.

In the bleak emptiness of the cover page and the eloquence of her essay,
Dr. Southgate uses the theme of art—visual, musical, and literary—to
forcefully depict the terrible loss and destruction humanity has suffered
because of HIV/AIDS.

Each week *JAMA* also includes both an original poem and a personal
essay whose subject matter relates to medicine. "Pulse," which is printed
once a month throughout the academic year, is a section of the journal
authored and edited by and for medical students. "Pulse" publishes student
writing (including poetry, essays, and fiction), research, and artwork. This
student section also prints the results of the annual William Carlos Williams
poetry contest, an event sponsored by a consortium of medical schools. In
the pages of *JAMA* I could witness how physicians are using the medium of
art to explore the meaning of their profession and their experiences as men
and women who daily come into contact with the most elemental, inescap-
able truths which define the human condition—birth, illness, recovery,
death, and suffering.

Throughout that fall of 1990 and into the winter and spring of 1991,
I became increasingly involved in researching the relationship between
medicine and literature, bringing my personal background to my work. I
also became more immersed in the medical world as my health continued
to decline. Over time, the two aspects of my life, my illness and my work,
grew more intertwined, each giving me insight into the other. I derived
great satisfaction from my studies for their own sake, but my explorations
in the area of medicine and literature served, too, as a way to create meaning and sense out of all I was observing and experiencing in the world of
illness.

Over the months, Dr. Averapporti and I continued in our struggles to
control the lupus, or at least contain it. Of most concern to both of us
were the neurologic symptoms. My gait was changing. I was favoring one
side, limping and dragging one foot. I walked with a wider base of support
to compensate for difficulties with balance. I was losing more sensation in
my legs. In both my hands and legs, I felt tingling and pins-and-needles.
My limbs, especially my extremities, were becoming weaker. Headaches
were a constant problem.

But the exact origin of the neurologic problems was still a mystery. In December 1990 Dr. Averapporti sent me to a neurologist after I had several episodes during which I almost fainted. My vision blurred, and I had violent shakes. I felt nauseous, weak, and disoriented. I had trouble keeping my balance. One especially frightening attack occurred while I was on the subway. Philadelphia's public transportation system is old, dirty, and decrepit. I lurched through the dank, foul tunnel to the steep, unevenly worn stairs. I stumbled my way slowly, unsurely up to the daylight. Several people asked if I needed help. When I finally made it to the top, I almost fell backward down the flights of stairs behind me. Fortunately I caught the rail in time. Out on the street, I found a bench, rested awhile, then caught a cab back to the dorm.

Instead of seeing a neurologist at CGH, I decided to see the one who had cared for various members of my family. After an initial examination and several nerve conduction tests, he decided that I had peripheral neuropathy. He reassured me that I did not have any central nervous system disease, in other words, no involvement of the spinal cord or brain.

Dr. Averapporti continued his attempts to control the disease and ease my symptoms. We increased the steroids, but the disease would not yield. Finally Dr. Averapporti decided that I should be hospitalized for pulse steroids.

That hospitalization marked a turning point for me in my relationships with my physicians. During that academic year, the wounds left by previous physicians had begun to heal. Dr. Averapporti, with his intelligence, compassion, and kindness, had been winning my trust. Our relationship had evolved into a partnership in which we made decisions about my treatment together. I found that this kind of doctor-patient relationship worked best for me. It was far better than the father-daughter interaction I had experienced with Dr. Kostos or the authoritarian style of Dr. Warner. I was equally impressed and reassured by the many specialists to whom Dr. Averapporti referred me. For the most part, they were a young, enthusiastic, smart, and understanding group, and not one physician was condescending, patronizing, or inept.

However, despite my growing security with my health-care professionals, I still panicked at the idea of a hospital stay, my fears setting off loudly pealing alarm bells in my mind. This would be my first hospitalization since the days of Drs. Kostos and Warner. What if Dr. Averapporti made me the scapegoat for my disease, as they had done? What if he abandoned me, leaving me to deal with this disease on my own?

But Dr. Averapporti did not disappoint me. Though every so often I still feel a twinge, an ache of doubt coming from the old wounds, especially at times when the cause of the disease activity is particularly hard to explain, after that hospital visit, my faith in Dr. Averapporti was firmly established. Out of that faith, in that fertile soil of peace and trust, there flowered a kind of healing.

I have come to you
in the shadowy realm of dreams
when sleep was restless,
filled with pain I brought with me
from my waking hours.
No peace to be found in
my tortured night.

I lay on the gurney,
consumed by fierce fire flames;
I called out your name.
You appeared by my side,
white coat rustling softly.
You took my hand in yours,
locked your gaze with mine,
and said,
"All will be well.
Quiet, untroubled sleep
will be yours through this night."
With your hand still touching my own,
you stayed until
I drifted away to a place where
pain did not follow.

I awoke the next morning,
feeling refreshed and soothed,
the dream still vivid.
I was puzzled.
At least in my daylight hours,
I know that you are not an
all knowing angel of the night
but a man of flesh and blood
who has confessed to me

the uneasiness of his sleep
sometimes,
when his powers to heal
seem all too limited,
the tools at his command
slippery serpents who could slither
out of his grasp,
then poison, destroy.
Yet the serpents can also carry
health's nectar in their sharp fangs.
With a sigh and a prayer,
you use the serpent.
But it sometimes sits coiled in your dreams,
mocking you, taunting you
with all its uncertainties.

All this I know—
no mystical power
in your hands, your eyes.
I have read the studies,
seen the statistics.
I am a child of science,
raised on facts and logic,
trained, like you,
to understand physical relief
as a result of the knife
or the pharmacy.
Magic, in its way, one might say,
but certainly not the product of dreams.
I do not believe
in shamans.

Perplexed, I put the dream aside.
We spoke with precision of blood counts
you and I, in your gleaming,
antiseptic, examining room.
Then, one night, as I tossed and turned,
trapped in molten bars of pain,
I called out once more.
You answered.

What have I seen in your office,
with your bookshelves heavy with texts
overflowing with modern scientific knowledge?
What have I heard in your voice,
weighty with the authority of technology?
Did I hear the chant of the priest,
sense the healing ritual of ages past,
from a time before Microbiology?
Perhaps I just felt the force of your compassion,
mingled with my own faith and hope.

I do not know,
yet I have come to accept these dreams,
these nocturnal encounters infused
with a magic and mystery
which cannot be explained by dissection,
nor understood through the microscope.
When we meet in the daytime,
we will speak of
serpents, scans and white cells.
But in the deepest of night,
it is your eyes and your touch
which will bring me comfort and relief,
the powers of night and day
joined together in an effort to heal,
creating a whole,
interknit.

The academic year was almost at an end. When I reflect back upon it, I think of that year as a time of pervasive physical illness. But I remember it, too, as a time of emotional healing under Dr. Averapporti's care. Also, during that year, my way of handling my illness changed. I still compartmentalized my life to a certain extent, trying to keep some separation between my illness and what I considered my normal routine of social and school activities. I entered CGH's doors and, by turning on a mental switch, I assumed the role of patient. I walked out the door, pressed another switch, and became Melissa again—student, writer, researcher, family member, and friend. But the division between my two existences was no longer so rigid. I did not leave Melissa, with all her individuality, outside CGH. I brought my interests, experiences, and talents to my interactions with my health-care professionals, and I used my encounters in the hospital to illuminate, inspire, and guide my academic research.

By making the line of demarcation between my "illness life" and my "regular life" more fluid, I found that each part benefited the other. By sharing our love for writing, the health-care professionals and I had found a special way to connect. As a participant observer, I had studied with great excitement the powerful role that creative writing was playing in the medical community. Literature was not just material for academic analysis; it lived as a vital, active force in the world of medicine. My experiences gave my commitment to writing a new depth and meaning. There in the desert sands, I was finding a path that I could truly call my own.

13

Land of the Midnight Sun

Summer 1991

IN THE middle of April, just before the end of that academic year, my friend Michael, who also lived in Washington House, was in my room playing with my contraband kitten, Dickens. I had met Michael in my freshman year of college, and our friendship had quickly grown. He was a dual major in both mathematics and business. He was extremely intelligent, analytical, and, like Dickens, insatiably curious. The questions Michael put to people were blunt almost to the point of rudeness. But I soon learned that his queries were never malicious. He was just incredibly honest about what he thought and what he wanted to know. In fact, he possessed a generous, caring, and kind heart. In many ways he was an idealist, though he would have scoffed at this description, preferring to think of himself as a tough realist. He actively participated in volunteer efforts in ghetto neighborhoods in the city. After college Michael wanted to work for a nonprofit organization, though his mother was vehemently opposed to the idea. She felt that he should pursue a high-paying, secure job in the for-profit sector. I wondered who would win the battle.

Not only were Michael and I close, but he had also gotten to know my family. He often visited my home in Maryland. On one of his later visits, he dropped his bag in the foyer, sighed, and said, "Now I'm home." He felt so comfortable in my parents' house that he proceeded directly upstairs to what he called "his room" (the guest bedroom), scooping up his favorite cat along the way to keep him company while he unpacked.

That April day, Michael and I were sitting in my dorm room talking about our plans for the summer. I would be staying with my family in

Maryland for the vacation. He was going to Sweden with his mother to spend time with his mother's family. His mother, Ms. Peterson, and her two sisters, were born and raised in Sweden, on a farm in the rural outskirts of Stockholm. Michael's mother had met his father while he was traveling through Sweden. They married, and her husband brought her to New York, where Michael grew up. By the time Michael was in college, however, his parents had been divorced for some time. Ms. Peterson's family had kept the farm. Her sisters, both single, went to the country on the weekends and holidays. During the week, each sister lived in her own apartment in Stockholm. Michael's aunts were nurses.

Michael was in the middle of describing the country home and his aunts when he interrupted himself and exclaimed, "Why don't you come with me?" I was taken completely by surprise. I was immediately excited by the idea and flattered by the offer, but I was hesitant to accept. "Michael, thanks for inviting me. It sounds wonderful. But don't you think you should consult your mother and your aunts? They don't see you that much, and they might not be thrilled about me intruding on your time together. How about you discuss it with your family, and I'll ask my doctor what he thinks." Michael spoke with his mother that night, and she called her sisters. They told Michael that they would be happy to have me stay with them.

I scheduled an appointment with Dr. Averapporti before I left school. I asked, "Dr. Averapporti, how would you feel about my spending three weeks in Sweden? I would be leaving in the middle of June." Dr. Averapporti approved the trip, though it was with some misgiving. "Melissa, I'd prefer you to be in better health before you travel. But you're the one who has to know your own limits: if you feel that you can physically handle the trip, then that has to be your decision. But you must go with the right attitude. You can't tour until you drop. You must pace yourself." He advised that if I did not feel well while I was away, I should raise my steroid dosage.

Dr. Averapporti and I also talked about my neurologic symptoms, which continued to be of particular concern to both of us. I was experiencing great difficulty with what is known as a "foot drop." My right foot was very weak, and I had trouble picking it up. Often it would catch on uneven surfaces, causing me to trip and sometimes fall. Dr. Averapporti referred me to the orthotics department so that I might be fitted for a brace that would prevent my foot from dragging.

I explained to the orthotist that I would be leaving for Sweden in a few weeks and needed the brace by then. The orthotist promised that he would have it ready for me, and he did. The brace was a milky-white, lightweight plastic. It extended across the bottom of my foot and up my ankle, covering the back and sides of my calf to the knee. Under the brace, I wore a thick sock made especially for the orthotic. The brace was kept in place by a velcro strap at the top of the orthotic.

The brace was definitely helpful; it held my foot at a ninety-degree angle to my leg, keeping the foot out of my way. Walking became much easier. But at first I felt awkward and self-conscious. The brace invited questions; it transformed my disease into a visible entity. When people asked why I was wearing a brace, I usually quickly explained, "Oh, I have problems with my back that affect my foot." Then I changed the subject. When I came to know a person better, I gave more information.

My disease had been highly visible the year before, while I was undergoing rehabilitation, but at that time the physical therapists and the physician viewed my physical deficits as temporary. Wheelchair, walker, assorted crutches, and canes were seen merely as tools to be used until I fully recovered. This attitude made it easier for me to deal with needing the adaptive equipment. Now my situation was different. I was told that my foot drop could heal, but my doctor could not give me a guarantee. He could also not tell me how long I would need the brace. My foot drop was seen as part of a chronic rather than an acute process. Because of the uncertainty and the potential for long-term use, I found it hard to accept the brace.

Having the brace also meant that I was limited in the kinds of shoes I could wear. I needed a shoe that tied or came up high enough on the foot to grab hold of the brace. I had loved pretty shoes, and I had at least half a dozen flats in all different colors to match my outfits. Because of my precarious balance, I had given up high heels some time ago, but I still could manage low heels. With the brace, I could no longer use the flats and the heels. I boxed the shoes up and put them in the closet, anticipating the time when I could wear them again. They are in that box still. Though it has been five years, I cannot bring myself to throw them away. For that box contains more than shoes. It holds my hope that someday I will not need the brace. I see that box and hear the tap of my heels as I whirl around the dance floor, free and unencumbered, feeling attractive and feminine.

During those weeks before I left for Sweden, the neurologic symptoms intensified, and I lost more of my treasured independence. I was driving to the bank when a child darted onto the road. I was not going fast; I saw the little boy immediately, and I should have had plenty of time. I did manage to stop the car and avoid hitting the child. Just barely. My reflexes were slow, and I did not have enough strength in my foot to slam on the brakes. I drove slowly home, my body shaking—in fright, relief, and anger. I knew I was no longer fit enough to drive.

I pulled up in the driveway and shut off the car. I pulled the key out of the ignition and held the shiny metal in my palm, remembering the day I passed my driving test and received my license. The sense of exhilarating independence when I no longer had to rely on my parents to take me every place I wanted to go. Sixteen years old. An American coming of age. Now it was as if the clock were turning backwards, and I was a child. Helpless. Dependent. Needy. I left the car and entered the house. I placed my car keys in a drawer, not knowing when I would be able to use them again.

Fortunately I had little time to dwell on my physical state during those first few weeks of my summer vacation. Time seemed to vanish as I prepared for my trip. My family joined enthusiastically in my plans. Mom took me shopping for supplies. Dad rushed me down to Washington, D.C., so that I could receive my passport in time. Bubbe Pearl advised me on ways to keep my luggage light; since I would be traveling alone, I needed to be able to manage my own bags. My vacation turned into a family enterprise.

Finally came the day of departure. When, after a long flight, I arrived in Stockholm, Michael, his aunts, and his mother were at the airport to greet me. His aunts, Birgit and Signhild, did not speak any English, but their warm smiles and friendly manner made me feel welcome. We rode for about half an hour on a bus that transported us to the family's country home in Sigtuna. I was told that the bus stopped right at the house, but that was not exactly true. After the bus dropped us off, we had to walk about a half mile, cross a bridge, and go through a meadow to get to the house. There was no road or driveway, only grass. The meadow sloped steeply, and instead of a handrail, there were poles set a foot or so apart. I had one heavy suitcase (more than fifty pounds) and a tightly packed carry-on bag, but fortunately, Michael's aunts took my luggage. In fact, throughout the trip, they never let me carry my bags. I could not have managed without all their generous help.

We arrived at the house. The aunts took my luggage inside and gestured for me to sit on the glider in the garden. When they returned, they brought a tray of drinks and fruit. We relaxed and chatted. Michael and his mother translated for me and the aunts. After we all were rested and refreshed, we went inside.

The house was charming. It was a two-story frame house painted maroon. Shutters and trim gleamed white. To the right of the house as one faced the front door was the lake. To the left, opposite the lake, were magnificent gardens blazing with color—flowers in varying shades of oranges, peaches, yellows, lavenders, and reds. Plum, apple, and pear trees provided fruit for the family. The aunts grew beets, potatoes, peas, carrots, currants (red and black), rhubarb, strawberries, and raspberries. By the gardens, facing the water, were the glider, a table, and chairs. A wide expanse of lush green lawn separated the barn and the outhouse from the main house.

I had been warned before I came that there were no indoor bathrooms in the house. Chamberpots were kept under the bed for emergencies and at night. There was running cold water in the kitchen for washing dishes. But to take a bath, one had to heat water on the wood stove and wash oneself while standing in a large basin. Fortunately, there was a heat wave while I was there; the temperature soared into the upper eighties. This meant that it was hot enough for me to swim and bathe in the lake. I have pictures of me in a bathing suit standing among the lily pads, washing my hair.

The house was relatively small but cozy, filled with nooks and crannies. It was also absolutely immaculate. The first floor consisted of a kitchen, family room, and bedroom. The family room contained beautiful dolls and old photographs of the family. Plants and fresh flowers were everywhere, giving the room added color and life. On the second floor were three more bedrooms. I was given the bedroom on the first floor, because the aunts did not want me climbing the steep, narrow staircase to the second floor. My bedroom was quaint and welcoming. The brass bed was covered by a thick down quilt. A soft, padded armchair stood in one corner. The aunts had placed a bowl of fruit and a vase of fresh flowers on the marble-topped chest of drawers. Delicate lace curtains framed the window, which overlooked the lake.

Michael had explained my health problems to his family. They were so understanding and tactful, giving assistance when it was needed without being intrusive or overly solicitous. They knew about my many various dietary restrictions. Apparently, Signhild had haunted the local supermarkets looking for special foods I could eat.

At first I was embarrassed by Signhild's efforts on my behalf; I apologized to Michael's mother for putting Signhild to so much trouble. But Michael's mother said, "Signhild enjoys taking care of people. It gave her pleasure to do this for you. Please don't apologize." The oldest of the three sisters, Signhild was a motherly woman, affectionate yet quiet, unlike Birgit, who, though also warm and caring, was more feisty and outspoken. I realized that I would only hurt Signhild if I refused her gifts and gestures or let them make me feel uncomfortable. I reminded myself that there is a graciousness to receiving as well as giving.

But I did not want to just take from these people; I tried to offer my help where I could. It was not within my power to chop the wood, bring drinking water from the well, or perform other heavy chores around the farm, but I did set the table and dry the dishes. Actually, when I first picked up a dish towel after dinner, Birgit was scandalized. I was a guest, and according to Swedish rules of hospitality, I should not be doing any housework. However, I used the language barrier to my advantage and pretended not to understand. After a few days, we settled into a routine. As she washed and I dried, we attempted to communicate, mostly through gestures. I enjoyed the time we spent together, and I know that she appreciated my small efforts to contribute to the household work.

Michael and I spent a relaxing week in the country. We celebrated Midsummer's Eve, an important Swedish holiday. Birgit set up a six-foot maypole on the front lawn. Other family members came for dinner that evening to celebrate the occasion. In the twilight, we picnicked by the maypole. Before I went to bed, Signhild instructed Michael to tell me that on this special night, I must pick seven different wildflowers and place them under my pillow, as I would then dream of my future husband. In the night that fell as lightly as mist, I gathered my wildflowers. I smelled their sweet scent as I drifted off to sleep, and though I know I dreamt that night, I awoke not remembering any of my dreams, much to the aunts' disappointment.

At the end of the first week, Michael and I left for Stockholm; his aunts and mother remained in Sigtuna. Birgit gave us a key to her apartment, so we could stay there while we toured Stockholm for a week. I have many memories of that graceful city, known as the "Venice of the North," which consists of fourteen islands joined by fifty bridges, and many canals.

Though we visited many of the popular tourist attractions, as time went on, I felt more like a native. I was not staying at a hotel, but in a Swedish apartment. I even cooked dinners for Michael and me in Birgit's tiny kitchen. Michael had lived in Sweden as a child and had spent summers there ever since. He had dual citizenship; he considered himself both Swedish and American. He was completely familiar with the city and spoke Swedish fluently, without an American accent. He taught me some basic Swedish words. One day a street vendor motioned to me to come over. He spoke in Swedish, and while I did not understand his words, I knew that he was trying to sell me his wares. I answered, "Nein tak" (No thank-you). He responded in his own language, mistaking me for a Swede. I smiled, and Michael and I moved on. Michael laughed at me and said, "You're becoming more Swedish every day!" Michael and I took public transportation everywhere, moving about the city with ease. Because I was with Michael, I was not treated as a tourist. I found myself shedding my usual identity and becoming a part of everything around me in a way that would not have been possible if I had been traveling with non-natives. I had left my everyday self behind, including my illness; I felt young and free.

Michael was unfailingly considerate of me during the vacation. Each morning when we made our plans to go sightseeing, Michael called the palaces, museums, or other places we had chosen to visit and asked about elevators and the amount of walking involved in the tour. We scheduled our day to minimize the walking I would have to do. I never asked him to do any of this; my pride would never have allowed me to do so. I did wonder how he knew to think of these things. Later I discovered that our friends from college, specifically Teresa, Mary and Jessica, had taken Michael aside and given him very exact instructions. And they had threatened him with bodily harm if he did not deliver me back in the same state in which he had received me. So I am not sure if his solicitude stemmed from concern for my welfare or fear for his own!

Regardless, I was touched. And I do believe that he enjoyed my company, as I did his. Whenever we could not fit an activity into our day, Michael would say to me, "You'll just have to come back again another summer." He wanted me to tour the Norwegian fjords with him on my next trip. We grew much closer over those three weeks, our friendship deepening. I treasure his friendship still.

Though there were many sights that fascinated me, I particularly enjoyed my visit to Stockholm's City Hall, where the Nobel prizes are awarded. The ballroom, also known as "The Golden Hall," was spectacular. Its walls are decorated with mosaics depicting the history of Sweden. The thousands of tiles are made of gold set in glass.

At the end of that week, Ms. Peterson and Birgit joined Michael and me in Stockholm. From there, we all boarded the Inlands Banan (Inland Railroad). We headed north, through Lapland, past the Arctic Circle. Again the family anticipated my needs. The sleeping car had three bunks, one on top of the other. Ms. Peterson and Birgit insisted on taking the higher bunks so I would not have to climb the ladder. Poor Birgit slept badly on the topmost bed, where the air was close and stuffy.

During the day, from the large picture windows, I watched the passing scenery with great interest. We rode for hundreds of miles without seeing any evidence of human habitation. There were thickly wooded forests, dense and dark with towering trees. They seemed timeless, ageless, enchanted. I was reminded of all the fairy tales I had read as a child—Hansel and Gretel, Little Red Riding Hood, and Snow White. The tour guide told us that trolls were said to live in the forests. I could believe it.

We passed by large lakes lying peacefully at the base of the mountains. There were also rocky expanses marked by huge boulders. Only a few stunted trees dotted the landscape. Glaciers had created these fields of stone and carved out the sharp peaks of the mountains. The hand that shaped the Swedish countryside on the outskirts of Stockholm was a gentle craftsman. Yet I preferred the jagged beauty of these regions near the Arctic.

I also took great pleasure in seeing the animals. The forests were filled with bears and reindeer. The reindeer often crowded on the train tracks, sunning themselves in the open space. The train would then have to stop until they cleared the path. At one point, we saw hundreds of reindeer, males with their great antlers as well as females and their young.

As the train carried me farther away, I think that a part of me almost believed that I could leave my illness behind. But my symptoms became worse as the trip progressed. At one stop toward the end of the day, I could not tour the village. The steps to get off the train were particularly steep there, and my balance, shakier than it had been when we set off from Stockholm, was not up to it. Even if I could have managed the steps, I was too exhausted to walk around. As we departed from the village, I looked into the forest and saw the wolf staring at me. I scowled at him fiercely, and he loped off into the woods, beyond my view. Though I could no longer see him, I sensed his presence close by. But I was determined that he would not steal this experience from me.

We reached the Arctic Circle and continued several hundred miles beyond, where we stopped for two days in Gällivare, a small town. There we visited the local sights. Perhaps my favorite spot was a tiny Lapp church. The tour guide was Lapp, a young woman with a dark complexion, brown hair, and vivid green, almond-shaped eyes. She was stunning and looked to be at least partly Asian. From her home in the mountains, fifteen miles away, she walked to work. Her family herded reindeer. Apparently, it was common for the men to stay behind with the herd while the women worked in town.

The church was 250 years old. It was a simple wooden structure, not ornate like the cathedrals we had seen in Stockholm. Yet to me, this place possessed a dignity and a raw beauty that made it outshine its urban counterparts. Set on the altar of rough-hewn wood was a weathered wooden sculpture of two men praying as they knelt in front of a log. I pictured the men talking to a personal God, speaking to Him as they sat beneath a tree in one of the forests He had created, a log their only altar. I felt a peace settle upon me. Though I knew not to whom or what I spoke, I added my own prayer to the silent words of the two men, and in that humble, holy place, I sensed a listening presence.

I asked to be brought safely through this trip, for my physical state was deteriorating, and fatigue and pain were washing over me in waves. I would think that I could not go any further, but then the tide would turn, and the waves would recede, allowing me to set forth again.

Perhaps God was watching over me. Or perhaps my surges of energy might be attributed to Birgit's Swedish remedy, which consisted of infusions of chocolate. She kept a constant supply of the richest chocolates on hand, and when I would begin to go pale and start dragging, she would administer some "medicine" from the box to renew my strength and give me energy. Out of all the treatments I have undergone, I must say that Birgit's is my plan of choice!

On our last night in Gällivare, we went up a mountain to see the midnight sun, an often elusive sight for it hides behind clouds and rain the few days a year it appears. At 11:30 P.M., the taxi carried us up the mountain to the spot with the best view.

The night was clear and cloudless, the patches of snow sparkled in the sun, which burned with a noontime intensity. Below us lay Sweden, rich shadings of green and blue, visible to us for a hundred miles in several directions. Slowly, the sun descended in the sky but never disappeared below the horizon. I remember how the penetrating stillness was filled with a delicate, soft light that was not extinguished even as the night continued onward. We were all awed by that sight. Ms. Peterson clasped my hand. In a hushed voice she said, "Did you ever think you'd be able to come here? No one will believe you when you tell them everything you've done and seen—despite your illness." We all stood together on the mountaintop, and that became the epitome of hope for me. Night lit by sunlight, an act of God I was able to witness through the love and friendship of family and friends.

We came back from the Arctic and spent a few more days in Stockholm before returning to the country home. I will never forget the dinner cruise we took one evening. We sailed out to a string of islands in the Baltic, an archipelago of twenty-four thousand wooded and rocky islands, some inhabited, others untouched. The ship was elegant and stately. Built in 1912, it was the oldest passenger ship still in use. During dinner, a formal, gourmet meal, we sat with an older Swedish couple. Their English was superb, and we had a delightful conversation. They advised us about the sights we must not miss while in Stockholm, and we talked about Swedish politics and customs. They pointed out their villa, which we could clearly see from our window.

After dinner we docked at one of the islands, where we listened to a French horn and harp concert in an old palace. The palace needed restoration, but it still retained its regal air despite its shabbiness. Its faded beauty spoke of ages past and gave it a poignancy that blended with the mournful, melodic tones of the music. As we listened, we watched the sun go down and twilight settle over the performers, who played in front of windows overlooking the sea. In the same moment, the last of the light and the final notes of the music disappeared into the night. We boarded the ship once more and returned to Stockholm.

I spent the last five days of my vacation in the country. During that time, my parents as well as Bubbe Pearl and Zaide called me. My other grandparents sent me a card, and I received a letter from Minh. Michael's family thought this was hilarious. I had left home for only three weeks. But my family and friends were thinking of me and wanted to know how I was doing.

One day after I had been in contact with my family, Ms. Peterson and I were sitting outside in the glider, my special spot. We talked about my close relationship with my family. Her eyes teared as we spoke. Was she thinking of her mother, who had died five years before? Or was she feeling the pain of being separated from her family in Sweden? Ms. Peterson then confided that Michael was lonely for their family in Sweden. As a result of the divorce, Michael did not see his father or his father's family often, and Ms. Peterson felt that Michael cared so much for his friends because he was trying to replace the extended family he yearned for.

Ms. Peterson's words settled deep into me as we sat in silence, rocking slowly back and forth on the glider. For so long I had been ashamed of the increasing dependence on others that the illness forced upon me. Guilt was my constant companion, and I thought of myself sometimes as a parasite. But Michael's mother reminded me that I could still reach out to others in essential ways. Neither I nor any of Michael's friends could ever completely fill the absence of Michael's family. But through my friendship I could offer him the support and caring he so needed and wanted. My illness did not have to stop the natural flow of giving and receiving upon which I had built my relationships with friends and family, the connections and ties that created the structure and meaning in my life. In the distance I saw the wolf once more, briefly, before he disappeared into the fields, his tail brushing the ground, his head held low. Defeated enemy.

The week ended, and it was time for me to head for home. As I said my good-byes to Michael and his family, I knew that I would miss the aunts and Sweden, a country I had embraced and which, I felt, had embraced me. Before I left, Signhild said to me, using Michael as a translator, that I should send my best wishes from her to my parents, and I must tell them that they should be very proud of their charming, wonderful girl. Her words meant so much to me. In spite of the language, culture, and illness barriers, I had formed a connection with this kind woman and her family.

By the time I boarded the plane, the lupus was flaring out of control. I was barely able to walk. I needed wheelchair assistance. I was one solid, burning mass of pain from my head to my toes. My muscles were sore, stiff, and cramped. I felt as if a sharp knife were slicing through my back, laying it open to expose bare nerve and bone.

I was now numb from my waist to my toes. Before I left Sweden, I had rummaged through my suitcase looking for a pair of socks, but when I went to put them on, I saw to my surprise that I was already wearing socks. I stared at the white cotton. Without looking, I did not know the socks were on my feet. My hands and arms were also numb up to the middle of my forearms.

My limbs were strangers to me. I had odd sensations in my legs—tingling and burning, as well as the usual pins-and-needles. It seemed as if a tight band were wrapped around my legs. My legs and tremoring hands felt so heavy, clumsy, and weak. There were times, each episode lasting a minute or two, when my hands would become rigid and locked, turning into useless blocks of solid concrete. My hands and legs would jerk involuntarily. I was embarrassed when my right leg shot out into the aisle of the plane, nearly tripping a stewardess.

In addition to problems with balance and coordination, my vision was blurred, and I had pain behind the right eye. Dizziness was yet another symptom. I remember lurching toward destinations I could not clearly see, struggling to retain my balance as the ground seemed to ripple beneath me. All my other lupus symptoms were flaring as well: arthritis, sores in my mouth and throat, rashes, fevers, fatigue, Raynaud's, nausea, abdominal pain, diarrhea, reflux, loss of appetite, bladder problems, and shortness of breath.

When I got home I called Dr. Averapporti, and that day, I was in his office. He sent me directly to a CGH neurologist, Dr. Ominsky. From there, I was admitted to the hospital. The CGH neurology staff were unanimous in their diagnosis: I was suffering from myelopathy. "Myelopathy" is a general term for disease of the spinal cord. The CGH neurologists were shocked that the diagnosis had not been made earlier, particularly when I had experienced my first major myelopathic attack under Dr. Kostos's care eighteen months before.

Lupus rarely affects the spinal cord. Only one half of one percent, or one in two hundred, lupus patients have this type of involvement. My neurologic symptoms were similar to those of multiple sclerosis. The doctors debated. Was the myelopathy due to lupus or a separate disease process such as multiple sclerosis? In the end they decided that the question was one of academic rather than clinical interest; their method of treatment would be the same regardless of the ultimate cause. Steroids are the indicated treatment for an acute attack of myelopathy, so I was given IV pulse steroids for three days.

I finally had a label for the neurologic symptoms that had been a part of my disease almost from the beginning. But there was still a great deal of uncertainty. The doctors could not predict the course the disease would take or what further treatment I might need. They were also puzzled by one aspect of my clinical abnormalities. According to their physical examination, I should not have been able to walk at all. I certainly did not move with sureness or ease, but I could still totter about. Though a friend was appalled by what the doctors had told me, thinking it morbid and depressing, I was heartened. To me, the doctors' reaction indicated that I had more control over my physical state than they thought possible. And their remark was a source of comfort to me later. When the disease became more active, and doctors issued gloomy prognoses, I remembered that their knowledge was not absolute. It was important to be realistic, but I did not have to abandon hope.

I spent five days in the hospital, then returned to Maryland with my family. It was almost the end of July. I needed to recuperate and regain my strength before school began in September. The steroids did give me

some relief, but my neurologic deficits did not disappear. I mourned what
the disease had taken from me and wondered what the future would bring.
I was particularly frustrated with my awkward hands.

Some say the soul can be found
pulsing in the heart.
But I believe the soul resides
in our hands,
flowing through the grasping, nimble fingers
that separate us
from the kingdom of beasts
whose hearts beat like ours.
Towering pyramids,
tapestries of spun silver and gold—
all created by the work of our hands.

In the beginning
before words,
we spoke in fluid gesture.
Even now, though skilled artisans
in the craft of words
we still use hands to
emphasize a point, grace our speech,
saying, "I love you" in a gentle caress,
expressing anger and hate
in a curled fist.

I look down at my own hands made
stiff and clumsy by disease.
My fingers once spoke the language
of music as they danced over
keys of flute and piano.
As I look at my hands,
I realize they are empty.
My soul took flight,
traveled along the highways
of nerves and synapses
until it finally came to rest
at the source of all expression.

Though my hands are mute,
my soul reaches out in these words.
The silence is broken.

That summer was a time of coming to a new acceptance of my illness and myself, but it was also a time of broadening purpose. Once again I was studying with Esther, but now we had an additional goal for our work together. Esther had asked if I would be interested in co-creating and co-teaching a seminar with her based on our research in the field of medicine and literature. I had responded with an enthusiastic "Yes!"

My plans for the future had long included teaching, and now I would have the opportunity to see if it was something I really enjoyed. I would discover, too, if I had any talent for it. I had seen professors who considered teaching mere drudgery, a chore to be completed in order to pursue their research. The quality of their teaching reflected their attitude. I felt that these professors cheated themselves and their students. Everyone involved suffered. And if my illness had taught me anything, it was that my time and energy were too precious to waste on something I detested doing. University professors rarely teach before they enter graduate school and dedicate themselves to an academic career, so I greatly appreciated the unusual chance Esther was giving me. We spent the rest of the summer constructing our course, a freshman seminar, which we would be teaching that spring. We sorted through all our materials and decided that we would narrow our subject to the physician as writer.

Eventually, the summer came to an end. It was time to return to the university. As I looked ahead to my future, I saw the shadows cast by the wolf. But darkness did not engulf the landscape, for it was still lit by friendship, love, hope, and work. Day in the midst of night. So I journeyed on.

14

Destinations

Fall 1991–Spring 1992

THE SEASONS turned again; another school year had begun, my last as an undergraduate. As always, I quickly became absorbed by my school life. Esther and I continued to plan our seminar, and I began work on my senior honors thesis. I researched my topic under the direction of Dr. Philip Dawson, a professor in the English department, and Esther. As the months passed, Philip became both a friend and a mentor. I chose to write about William Carlos Williams—a prolific and important physician-writer. He practiced for more than forty years as a full-time general physician in the small town of Rutherford, New Jersey. He also specialized in pediatrics. Many of his patients were the poverty-stricken immigrants who lived nearby in Paterson, New Jersey.

Though many people in Rutherford knew him only as the "baby doc," during his lifetime Williams produced some six hundred poems, four full-length plays, an opera libretto, fifty-two short stories, four novels, a book of essays and criticism, his autobiography, a biography of his mother, an American history, a book of letters, a translation of a medieval Spanish novel, as well as several works that cannot easily be categorized within any one genre. Williams made a major contribution to literature. He and others of his generation yanked the poem out of the clutches of the remote, faded past and brought it into the hands of the modern age, irreversibly transforming the poem as well as the other genres of literature.

I was captivated by Williams, the man and his work. The force, power, and raw beauty of his poetry especially drew me to him. I was particularly fascinated with the ways that his identity and role as a physician, in terms of his scientific training and his medical practice, shaped his writing—his subject matter, style, and revolutionary literary theory.

I spent the next few months deep in the world of William Carlos Williams. In him, I found a kindred spirit. He wrote about his daily, lived experiences—in his case, as a physician, father, husband, neighbor, and friend. He, too, used his writing as a way to find and affirm the beauty, order, and meaning in a universe that so often seemed ruled by the chaos, suffering, and ugliness he witnessed on a regular basis. Writing was a way for him to form a connection to other people. Williams conceived of literature as a way for human beings to share their different worlds and become enriched by the exchange. Throughout his lifetime he was driven by an ethic of writing fundamentally tied to his ethic of living. As a physician, he played an integral role in the life of his community, and through his writing, he sought to tie himself even more closely to the world surrounding him. Writing was never an escape from the teeming world of ordinary humanity; on the contrary, Williams's writing bound him more closely to all those with whom he came into contact.

I thought of Williams in comparison to Oliver Sacks, a popular physician-writer and the author of *Awakenings* (made into a movie starring Robin Williams and Robert DeNiro). During our first summer internship, Esther had asked me to read Sacks's *The Man Who Mistook His Wife for a Hat,* a well-known collection of medical tales in which Sacks describes the bizarre neurologic disorders of various patients he treats. Esther did not offer her opinion of Sacks's work before I read his stories, but later she asked me what I had thought. I hesitated before answering. I assumed that she had assigned Sacks's work because she admired it. I, however, found his writings repulsive. Actually, so did she, but she did not want to bias my opinion; she wanted me to judge for myself.

I felt that Sacks presents his patients as nothing more than carnival freaks, and I received the impression that he places himself far above these oddities of nature whom he showcases. It also seemed to me that Sacks uses his patients' abnormalities in order to display his own superiority and intelligence. In a story about two idiot-savant brothers, Sacks proudly demonstrates that he is the only one brilliant enough to understand how the brothers communicate with each other through a language consisting of prime numbers. It is obvious that Sacks considers himself quite the math prodigy. Unlike Williams, who used his writings to bring him closer to others, Sacks employs his pen as a way of elevating himself above both his patients and his readers. For Sacks, literature becomes a way of removing and distancing himself from people. In this, Sacks goes against all I believe literature can and should be and do.

The beginning of the school year was an exhilarating time. I was filled with such excitement about my research. I am afraid my friends and family must have tired of Williams's name, so constantly did I make mention of him in those days. But that September was also a period of increasing disease activity. All the neurologic symptoms I had experienced over the summer became more severe, and a few new symptoms appeared. I was losing more sensation. The numbness crept upward from my waist and settled a few inches above, and the sensation loss that began in my hands extended past the elbow. My face felt stiff, and my smile had become lopsided. All my muscles had weakened; I even had trouble sucking liquid through a straw. I had problems swallowing. I often choked, and food seemed to get stuck on the way down.

My hands, increasingly rigid and stiff, also tremored more than ever. I am right handed and, unfortunately for me, the right hand was worse. My handwriting became atrocious. It was extremely difficult to take notes in class. Because I could not write quickly or legibly enough, I began to use a tape recorder for lectures. Even basic tasks like managing utensils were a challenge. My position sense was distorted. I could not tell where my hands and feet were located without looking at them. I might think that my hand was on my pillow when it was actually down by my side. My gait was slow and unsteady, and I began to drag the left foot, the one without the brace. Navigating the city streets was a difficult endeavor. I found myself continually late for class because I underestimated the time I needed. All my other lupus symptoms were flaring, too.

I was alarmed, not only by the symptoms themselves, but by how quickly they were intensifying. In the past, neurologic changes had been more gradual. It took at least a few weeks for me to spiral downward. Now I seemed to be falling, falling, all within a matter of days. I called Dr. Averapporti. At the end of September he put me into the hospital where I stayed for the next week.

It was during this hospital visit that we thought seriously about trying IV pulse cytoxan. Dr. Averapporti and I both wrestled with the question of whether or not to use cytoxan, and I think the decision was as wrenching for him as it was for me. The lupus was running rampant in my body. Cytoxan, one of the most potent immunosuppressants used in the treatment of lupus, *might* bring the lupus under better control, and, if it worked, we *might* also be able to decrease my steroids and minimize their side effects. But there were no guarantees, only uncertainty for us both.

A few years before, the National Institutes of Health (NIH) had set up a protocol for the use of cytoxan in patients with lupus nephritis, or kidney disease caused by lupus. At that time kidney disease was the focus of lupus research. Kidneys are well-understood organs. It is easy to measure kidney function and therefore evaluate the efficacy of various drug regimens. But central nervous system (CNS) disease activity is much harder to quantify—which makes it more difficult to study. NIH had issued no protocols, and no documentation for use of cytoxan in lupus patients with CNS disease. Would my type of lupus respond to the drug? What would the appropriate dosage be? How frequently should it be given, and how long should we continue the regimen? Dr. Averapporti had no studies to guide him.

Dr. Averapporti and I also had to deal with the important issue of cytoxan's many possible side effects. Cytoxan is a form of chemotherapy. Hair loss is common. Cytoxan can cause cancer. There is a significant risk of hemorrhagic cystitis, or bleeding from the bladder. Because cytoxan suppresses the immune system, the body becomes more susceptible and less able to fight infection. Cytoxan can cause ovarian failure and induce early menopause.

Of all the side effects that might occur, this last one worried me the most, much to my surprise. I was only twenty-one, more preoccupied with finishing college and pursuing my doctorate than marrying and starting a family. But when faced with the possibility of never giving birth, I realized the emptiness and grief I would feel if I were unable to bear children. I had not even known that this need was such a basic part of me. Premature menopause carried other powerful meanings; I associated it with the loss of my youth and femininity.

On several occasions, Dr. Averapporti and I spoke at length about cytoxan, its risks and benefits. He had sworn, as a physician, to above all do no harm. Treating me with cytoxan meant injecting me with a medicine toxic to my cells, a kind of poison, in order to quiet the lupus. Dr. Averapporti feared the consequences of his actions should we proceed with the chemotherapy. What if, by giving me cytoxan now, he condemned me to death by cancer ten or twenty years later? But at this point the lupus frightened him more. He felt the gamble was worth it.

I talked everything over with my parents. But in the end the decision had to be my own. I chose the cytoxan.

It was the day the cytoxan was to be given. The orders were written; it would be administered in a few hours, in the early afternoon. During his morning rounds, Dr. Averapporti came in to check on me. He stayed at the far end of the room near the door. He stood on one long leg which he jiggled slightly; the other leg he bent at the knee, foot flat against the door. He reminded me of a seabird on the sand, caught by an incoming wave and anxious to fly away to safer ground.

Before he escaped, I asked, my voice tremulous, my eyes not quite meeting his, "Do you think I'll ever be able to have children?" His body tensed, then stilled. He walked over to me and pulled up a chair beside my bed. Sitting very close to me, his body loose and relaxed, he spoke honestly but reassuringly about the chances and risks of my becoming pregnant and giving birth. I slowly calmed. He could give me no certainties, but he could offer me the sum of his knowledge and, most of all, the support of his understanding presence. He gave my hand a gentle squeeze, and then departed, no longer a bird in flight, but my physician and my partner who overcame his own fears, pain, and guilt to act as a friend and healer.

After Dr. Averapporti left, I dozed. Each time I came awake, it was with the overwhelming feeling that something awful was about to happen. Then I would remember. Cytoxan. Chemotherapy. While I was lying there, waiting, wondering, and worrying, my roommate's family walked in. I averted my eyes. I did not want to speak with anyone at that moment.

> Gathered before her small sleeping form
> her family surrounded her in an arc of love,
> and he—the deacon—filled the center.
> She lay before them, grown woman,
> yet childlike in her pain-filled vulnerability,
> submerged in the silence of narcotized dreams
> broken only by her occasional moan,
> the fleeting awareness of her broken body.
>
> I watched the tableau,
> detached,
> lost in my own world of chronic disease,
> the guardrails of my bed like prison bars,
> keeping me in and others out,
> the white sheets and blankets wrapped
> round me like a shroud

speaking to me of a dying,
the loss of the life I once knew.

I closed my eyes and began to drift,
hoping to find the release of sleep,
when out of the stillness came
words of prayer.
The deacon began,
calling upon Jesus Christ
to bless us both,
the woman and me,
who were in need of his healing.

Born under David's star
I bear no love for Jesus,
merely a man to me,
a legend, a mystic.
Yet as the deacon continued,
his words, his loving wishes,
spoken in a voice resonant, deep, and calm,
shattered the isolating wall of my illness.
Released from pain, my spirit joined them
as the arc closed and became a circle.

The hours passed more smoothly and swiftly after that. I now felt that I had the strength to receive the chemotherapy, the gift of healing poison. The treatment began. I was given medicines to make me comfortable. Though I felt mildly nauseous and my body ached as if I had the flu, nothing catastrophic happened. My hair did not suddenly fall out. As the nurse disconnected the IV, I felt an overwhelming sense of relief that it was over. I had come through.

During that hospital stay I was sent to physical therapy and occupational therapy. Arrangements were made for these two groups to follow me as an outpatient. In physical therapy, I was given a four-pronged cane, which I used over the next several months before graduating to a straight cane. The occupational therapist, who specialized in hands, fashioned splints for both of mine. After my discharge, I also returned to the orthotist, who made a brace for my left foot.

My disease was more visible than ever. Equipped with cane, braces, and splints, I received many stares and questions as I limped around the campus. It especially bothered me when some people would fix their gaze on the braces. They never saw *me;* all they saw was a pair of braces. Sometimes I dealt with these people by smiling at them, forcing them into direct eye contact. I hoped to make them acknowledge that there was a person wearing those braces. Most of the time, people did respond, and in their answering smiles, I felt less like an object, a mere piece of plastic.

In those autumn months, I dealt not only with how others perceived me; I also struggled with how I might see myself. Caught in the chaos of increasing disability and disease activity, grieving I searched for the essence of what defined me, my identity's core that illness could not reach. Then I reconstructed my self-conception based upon that essential, protected part of myself.

> Passing by the plate-glass window,
> I am arrested by a strange sight reflected there.
> It is a woman, young, in years,
> her body distorted by illness.
> She is pale except for sharp color in her cheeks,
> not the vigorous flush of youth
> but the stigma of disease.
> As I move past the store,
> she follows,
> moving slowly, painfully,
> one leg dragging stiffly behind.
> Her hair should be snowy white,
> her face wrinkled,
> bearing testimony to a full, long life.
> But her hair is not yet even gray,
> her face unlined and smooth.
>
> There is little youth in her body,
> yet there is vitality in the soul
> yearning to fuse itself with muscle and sinew.
> Then, once more, could the body allow the soul
> such exquisite pleasures as
> dancing to music's pulsing, insistent beat or
> walking to the constant rhythm of dreams unbounded—
> undarkened and whole.

I see the raw pain of this soul
still possessing in abundance
the grace and agility of youth
yet unable to connect with the clumsy body
acting as an inept and insensitive host
to its vibrant guest.

I feel anger and sorrow for this woman,
her spirit and body so grossly mismatched.
But as I look ever deeper into her eyes,
I am shaken by the power, strength, and beauty
of that entrapped spirit.
I find myself drawn to it.
I think,
I can love this woman.

I have come to the end of the storefront.
I journey a step further;
then the image disappears from view.
I feel an inner peace settle on me
gentle as the brush of a wing on a leaf
or the rustle of a soul.

That academic year was a constant round of doctors, therapy, and treatments. I was given IV cytoxan approximately once a month. A few days before the cytoxan, I would go to CGH's laboratory for pre-cytoxan blood work; ten days after each treatment, I needed to have blood drawn again. On the day of the infusion, I reported at eight in the morning to the short procedure unit (SPU). There I would remain for approximately the next nine hours. I was never afraid in the way that I had been the first time I received the chemo, and as the months passed, the treatments became part of my routine.

Becoming friends with the nurses helped me to make these chemo treatments a tolerable part of my life. When the nurses had free moments, they came to chat with me. We spoke about work, school, families, and our love lives. They were mostly young women only a few years older than myself. I came to know them well and consider them friends. Though I never looked forward to the treatments themselves, I did enjoy our conversations and appreciate the warmth and caring I found among these nurses.

I usually went to the SPU on a Friday, and my mother always made the drive from Maryland to be with me. When the treatment was over, she would take me to a nearby hotel, and then the next day, she would return me to my dorm room.

The first night after a cytoxan treatment was always the worst; I ached all over and just felt generally ill. For the next week, I dragged about as if I were suffering from the flu. But on the eighth day, the treatment's side effects subsided, to be replaced by overwhelming relief from the lupus symptoms. If I had the treatments on a Friday, by the following Saturday night, I felt renewed and filled with energy.

Even though I was learning to integrate these treatments into my life, the risk of premature menopause continued to haunt me. Each month, as the cytoxan coursed through the clear plastic tubing, I wondered if this would be the treatment that would take away my ability to have children.

> Though I try to keep
> ugly fear away,
> a stranger to my days,
> welcoming each hour
> without reservation,
> worries and doubts
> sometimes disturb
> my hard-won peace.
>
> As I traverse city streets,
> I carry my illness fears with me.
> My hand curved around
> the hard handle of the cane,
> braces wrapped around my legs,
> I wonder,
> Will I ever walk unaided, free?
>
> Once it seemed that the ability
> to move with ease and strength
> was my birthright,
> held over and given
> inalienably to me
> that day I took my first few steps.
>
> I allowed that perhaps
> when my hair turned snowy white,

but not before,
I might have to forfeit my right,
be as when I was first born,
dependent on others,
restricted.

There are treatments
which might keep my birthright
in my possession.
But this medicine could thieve
as viciously as the disease
by denying life
to my unborn children.
And is it not my right
to hold a baby of my own,
see my love between
myself and husband,
and all our ancestors
embodied in that
soft sweet child
cradled close to me?

Yet I have come to realize
that bearing children
or walking with
sure and steady steps
are only youth's customary gifts,
not incontrovertible rights.
Those gifts may yet be
bestowed upon me.
What a triumph, what a joy
will a stroll become
as my legs move in confidence and security.
How supremely delightful will be
my child's laughter.

Though fears sometimes ripple
through the calm waters
of my tenuous peace,
there are still places that fear

will never touch,
parts of me that illness
will never steal.

Though I may not be able
to give life,
I can always give
love
by sharing in the lives of those around me.
Dignity, love of others and self,
these I claim for my own,
inalienable rights,
completely untouchable.

I had come to accept the cytoxan; I was willing to endure the treatments, the side effects, and the risks, for its benefits. But it was always a difficult regimen, and I think it was as hard for my parents as it was for me. The monthly visits to Philadelphia physically exhausted my mother. She had to drive the 150 miles each way by herself. But the treatments also drained her emotionally. She hated the idea of my receiving chemotherapy. It terrified her. All the old feelings of guilt and helplessness surged through her once more. She told me years later that each month, after she dropped me off at my dorm room, she drove home weeping, feeling as if she were abandoning me.

My father was anxious, too. While I was undergoing the treatments, he stayed in Maryland in order to take care of the animals and hold down the home fort. But I know his mind and heart were with my mother and me. He worried about her driving when she was in such a distressed state, and of course, he was concerned about me. Each Friday and Saturday of my treatment were tense days for my father as he waited powerless by the phone to hear news of my mother and myself.

In addition to my monthly stays in the SPU, I visited the physical therapist three times a week and the hand therapist once a week. As in the past, therapists played very significant roles in my health care. Physical therapy again gave me a sense of control over my disease as I made a positive effort to overcome my physical disabilities. At the very least, physical therapy was a way to fight against losing more ground.

Besides the monthly trips to the SPU, the twice monthly lab work, the three visits per week to the physical therapist, and the weekly sessions with the hand therapist, I also regularly consulted with various doctors. I saw Dr. Averapporti at least once a month, and he still referred me to other specialists when he felt in need of their expertise. Sometimes I found myself at CGH three times in a week just to see physicians. By this point I greatly appreciated CGH's proximity to my dorm. I was able to integrate my complicated and time-consuming medical schedule into my daily routine only because I had no real commute to CGH. On my way to and from class and the library, I dashed into the hospital. Even with CGH's convenient location, it was still a challenge to fit everything into my life, my schoolwork, social activities, and medical appointments—all at a time when I was also dealing with so many physical symptoms, especially that persistent enemy, fatigue.

But when I pause a moment to reflect back on that academic year, the visits with various doctors, all the therapy, the treatments, and the flaring of my disease are not what I remember most clearly. What come to me are radiant memories of the life that stood apart from illness. I had been carefully tending my garden, and that year, the seedlings I had planted pushed through the earth and offered me their fragrant blossoms. I am thinking particularly of the spring semester I spent teaching with Esther.

Our freshman seminar, "Medicine and Literature: The Physician-Writer," met twice a week; each class lasted an hour and a half. For the first half hour to forty-five minutes, Esther or I would lecture to the students. After that we opened up the class for discussion. Though Esther and I both participated in guiding the discussions, each of us had her areas of expertise, and we divided up the lectures accordingly. My official position was that of a WATU (Writing Across the University) Fellow. I had been given a fellowship to teach the course as a writing-intensive seminar. This meant that each student was required to write at minimum three papers during the semester; at least two of the assignments were written in drafts.

The students turned in their first drafts to me. I critiqued the papers and met with the students individually for conferences about their writing. Esther also received a copy of the first drafts, and the students were given her written comments as well as my own, though Esther did not usually attend the meetings with the students. Esther and I marked the papers without consulting each other. When we were finished, we discussed each student's work. We always found that our assessments were in basic accord, a fortunate occurrence, because otherwise the students would have had to deal with conflicting advice.

From the beginning Esther made it clear to me and to the students that

I was more than a Writing Fellow: I was a co-teacher. Esther gave me a key to her office and placed my name and my office hours on her door. Because she felt very strongly that I was to be accorded the proper respect by the students, she felt that they should not call me "Melissa" and address her as "Dr. Stein." At first we tried asking them to call both of us by our first names, but it soon became evident that they did not feel comfortable using Esther's first name. They were too much in awe of her position as a well-known full professor. Because of my age, I seemed like a peer to them; they were more relaxed with me. Finally, by the middle of the semester the students resolved the problem themselves. Esther became "Dr. Stein" or "Professor Stein," and I, much to my amusement, was dubbed "Professor Melissa."

There were fifteen freshmen in the class. Most of them were planning to go to medical school but also had a keen interest in literature and writing. Some students used the class as a way to explore their future careers as physicians. Our course served as an accompaniment to the basic science courses they were all taking that year. Biology and chemistry gave them the science of medicine; we were introducing them to its art.

Though I taught these students more than four years ago, I still recall their names and faces, some of the startling papers they wrote, our writing conferences, and certain lively class discussions. These students were a pleasure to teach. Our course was not required. They were in our class because they were genuinely intrigued by the subject matter. Many professors shy away from freshman seminars, preferring to teach only upperclassmen or graduate students. But Esther did not feel that way. She had always enjoyed mentoring young people, and I could see why. These students were not jaded or blasé; they were eager and excited about what they were doing.

Our course was divided into ten topics. We started by reading *The Plague* by Albert Camus. Though Camus was not a physician, the novel is narrated by a doctor. Esther and I began the class with this book because it encompassed many of the themes we would discuss during the term. Next on our list were medical short stories. We assigned stories by William Carlos Williams and used an excerpt from Dr. Thomas Addis's *Glomerular Nephritis: Diagnosis and Treatment* in order to compare and contrast an actual case history with Williams's medical short stories. Esther and I continued to be fascinated by the artistic process, and we wanted to explore that topic with the class. Addis's work and Williams's stories shared much in common; many of Williams's pieces were taken directly from his actual experiences as a practicing physician. Yet there were fundamental differences between the stories and the case history. The stories were works of art, and the case history was not. Why? In what ways?

Our class discussions of Williams's work were some of the most heated of the semester. Many of the students were put off or even highly offended by Williams's seemingly insensitive and rude treatment of his poor, mostly immigrant patients. The stories we assigned came from a collection Williams wrote during the Depression. Overwhelmed and stricken by all the suffering he witnessed and was often powerless to relieve, he wrote the short stories partly as catharsis. He also hoped that through his frank, unrelenting and almost brutal portrayal of himself and his patients, he could shock his complacent middle-class audience into awareness of the poor's desperate circumstances. Through my extensive research of Williams and my exposure to much of his writings, I had gained a total view that the few short stories we read in class did not give. I was forced to leap to the defense of my literary hero, whose love for his patients, as well as his dedication to medicine and his work as a physician, are completely evident in his autobiography, his personal letters, and his creative writing.

Our other topics were entitled "The Symbolic Significance of the Human Body—Particularly the Human Heart," "Poetry," "The Essay," "Becoming a Physician: Initiation and Transformation," "A Questing Psychiatrist: Walker Percy, Religious Novelist," "The Doctor-Patient," "The Novel," and "Medicine, Media, and Pop Culture." Esther and I found that certain subjects sparked more discussion and interest than others. I was concerned about the students' response to the poetry, especially since I was one of the assigned authors. Much to my surprise, they were quite receptive, and we even spent an extra class session talking about poetry. Through the conferences I discovered that some of the students wrote poetry themselves. They were curious about my work and asked me many questions both in class and during our conferences. Because I had been willing to share my poems with the students, they felt comfortable giving their poems to me. Knowing that poetry is a deeply personal form I felt highly honored that they offered me their trust in this way.

Not every class was successful. I experienced the agony of lecturing to the class and finding that my questions were met with silence and glazed or confused eyes. During these sessions, time dragged with excruciating slowness. Esther and I would try to approach the material in ten different ways, and still there would be dead quiet. Our attempts to discuss Walker Percy were extremely unsuccessful. The majority of the students just did not have the background to read this physician-writer-philosopher, and they could not relate to his work. Esther and I decided that if we taught the course again, we would definitely drop Walker Percy from the syllabus.

I greatly enjoyed the class sessions, but I think I derived the most profound satisfaction and pleasure from the writing conferences. According to the terms of my WATU fellowship, I was required to spend only fifteen minutes with each student, but the conferences usually lasted at least half an hour, more often closer to an hour. It was a chance to really get to know the students. The student and I talked about his or her paper, but we also discussed his or her other classes, life at school, family, and plans for the future. Sometimes I was able to offer advice or assistance because of my own experiences or contacts at Laurel.

Students were assigned three papers during the semester. The first paper required the students to write a personal account of some illness experience or medically relevant event. It could involve a family member, a friend, a stranger, or the student. For the second paper, they wrote up an interview they had conducted with a health-care professional or a student training to enter the health-care profession. The last assignment was an analysis and discussion of patterns the student observed in the way that illness and medicine are portrayed in the media (newspapers, magazines, television, the movies).

Esther and I were moved and touched by many of the personal accounts. We felt privileged that the students had entrusted us with these narratives. A few papers especially come to mind. In one, "Hold My Empty Hands" the student, Linda, describes the devastating death of her grandmother. Linda was only eleven years old when her grandmother died. Linda was spending the day with her grandmother. They were watching television together, when her grandmother suddenly began choking on a piece of candy. Though Linda had been taught the Heimlich maneuver, in her panic, she could not remember the technique. She ran to the phone, then dropped it. She decided to get a glass of water, most of which she spilled as she dashed back to her grandmother. By this time, her grandmother had slumped to the floor, unconscious. Linda sat down beside her, begging her to drink the water, pleading with her not to die. Realizing that her grandmother was fading away, she went outside to find a neighbor, who then called 911. But by that time, it was too late.

That eleven-year-old child blamed herself for her grandmother's death; Linda had been carrying that child's burden of guilt for the past seven years. Before writing the paper, she had been unable to write or talk about the events of that terrible day. But in her eloquent, beautifully crafted essay, she was able to give voice to the pain she had held inside her. Writing brought her some healing and peace.

"The Grapefruit Bowl" was another essay I particularly recall. At least in the first draft, it was not that well done. The author of the paper, Scot, was not exactly a star pupil. He sat in the back of the room. With his slouched posture, eyes at half-mast, and his baseball cap pulled low over his forehead, his entire body language expressed supreme boredom and indifference. He rarely participated in the discussions. So, when he arrived to discuss his paper, which needed a great deal of work, I did not begin by being unkind or cruel, but I was not overly gentle, either.

Yet as the meeting progressed, I was astonished to find that the supercilious air and the apparent inattention were nothing more than a pose. He showed genuine concern about the paper. His piece was about the death of his grandfather. He truly cared about his grandfather and was extremely angry about the way in which his grandfather had been treated in his last days by the hospital physicians. The paper was very important to Scot. He wanted to communicate his love for his grandfather and his fury about the inadequacies of the medical care his grandfather had received. I even had trouble getting Scot to leave because he wanted to go over the paper in such detail. He genuinely wanted to learn how to make his points more effectively. When we also spoke about some of the assigned readings, I realized that he had been listening intently and forming his own opinions.

Scot's second draft was almost unrecognizable from the first, and the final paper was powerful and well-written. Scot continued to open up during our conferences, which gave me the chance to see the side of himself he kept hidden in class. His behavior in class never changed. But at least, through his writing and our meetings, I now knew that it was only a charade, though I never understood why he felt compelled to put on such an act.

The conferences really allowed me to get to know the students, and the class gave the students a chance to bond. I watched as some of them formed friendships that lasted throughout their college years. We all grew closer together after several people read their personal accounts to the class. One student, Lisa, made all of us teary eyed as she read aloud her paper in which she described her summer job as an emergency medical technician (EMT). One afternoon she was called to the scene of a suicide. The victim was a classmate from her high school. In her essay, Lisa struggled to make sense out of such a meaningless, tragic death.

In so many ways that semester, through student papers, writing conferences, and class discussions, I felt that I shared in the lives of my students. I also learned from them. My official role was that of their teacher, but I found that I was a student as well. The students brought their own perspectives to the literature. Our exchanges made me see the readings in a new light. When a student and I disagreed, I was forced to articulate my own opinions more clearly—and sometimes defend them. This kind of practice sharpened my critical skills. My writing gained strength from commenting on the students' work. I had to assess the strengths and weaknesses of their writing; I then became more aware when I was working on my own.

I learned, too, from Esther. I considered myself an apprentice in the art of teaching, a skill to be taught and cultivated. I have always thought that the academic system is flawed, because graduate students are thrown into teaching situations with little instruction. It is assumed that as long as the graduate student knows his or her subject, he or she will be an effective teacher. Just because someone is well educated in a particular field does not at all guarantee that he or she will be able to communicate their knowledge to students. That is entirely a separate ability. Esther and I met after each class in order to analyze the positive and negative aspects of that day's lecture and plan the next class accordingly. So, I learned through experience how to teach.

And there was something else that I learned that semester. I discovered the pleasures of writing in the fifth grade, when I wrote my first poem, the haiku about the eagle. As I grew older, that interest in writing became a vocation. Over the spring term, my sense of purpose broadened to include teaching. I was a writer, and I was a teacher. Both were ways to give to people and form vital, living links with them. Despite my illness, I still had something to offer others. I could fulfill the promise of my childhood. My illness had not taken that away.

During that year I began to feel an inner peace and serenity that flowed from my growing sense of purpose and direction. That sense of contentment was apparent to others. One day as I was walking on campus, a man stopped me and said, "I've seen you around the university." He gestured to my cane and braces and continued, "You obviously have problems, but you always look so happy. You have the most beautiful smile. I wish you the best of luck." Another time, a clerk at the local grocery where I shopped asked me, "You're always smiling. What's your secret?"

When people commented on my cheerfulness, I sometimes felt awkward. While it was true that I was finding genuine satisfaction and joy in my life, it was not as if I never felt sorry for myself, angry, worried, fearful, discouraged, or upset. But I had learned how to deal with my grief so that it would not consume me. I had decided a long time ago that though I could not control the physical disease, it was in my power to decide how to handle my illness. If I allowed the lupus to turn me into a bitter, self-pitying, self-centered person who could not take an interest in the life around her, then I would be permitting the lupus to change me into a person I did not want to be, someone I could not like or respect. This damage would be far more terrible than any scan or x-ray could ever measure.

But I did have my moments when the pain and losses of disease overwhelmed me, throwing me once more into grief's turmoil. There were two instances I especially remember from that year. In August, at my parents' urging, I had applied for Supplemental Security Income (SSI), disability payments from Social Security. My parents were in financial difficulties by this time; several publishers had reneged on book contracts they had with my father. He had been counting on those contracts. Though the publishers were in clear violation of the law, my father did not have the money to take them to court. My medical bills and general costs of my illness further strained my father's finances. I knew my receiving additional income would help lessen their burden, and I filed the papers without argument.

But I hated the idea of going on disability. I detested that label and all it implied. Though I realized that I did have significant physical limitations, I did not conceive of myself as handicapped. It also hurt my pride to think of taking handouts from the government. It is usually extremely difficult for lupus patients to get SSI; in fact, the Lupus Foundation of America periodically sponsors workshops to give lupus patients advice about how to apply for disability. I knew several lupus patients, some of them quite ill, who had been turned down. But after only a few months, Social Security notified me that I was eligible for SSI. I read the letter and cried. I wondered what kind of bleak picture my doctor had painted to have my application approved so (relatively) quickly and easily. I felt ashamed for receiving charity.

Eventually I was able to take a practical view. I needed the money. And, although being on disability meant that I fit into a certain category established by the government, it did not define *me*. I was not a useless or lazy person. I did have a future. This was a temporary situation until the disease came under better control. After I finished school, I would head into academia, support myself, and be financially independent.

I was also deeply discouraged that year when I was discharged from physical therapy in the middle of March. I was still using a cane and the braces, though I was no longer wearing the hand splints. The physical therapist decided that we had reached a plateau. Unless the disease quieted down, we could go no further. She told me that I needed to accept that some of my problems might be the result of permanent damage to my spinal cord and gave me exercises to continue at home. She said that because I was so physically active with all my walking and swimming, she was not worried about my getting enough exercise. She was more concerned that I conserve my energy.

To me, physical therapy had always represented hope that I could reverse the effects of the disease. Now I wondered if I would ever be able to walk without the cane and braces. Would I never dance, play a game of tennis, drive a car again? Would my condition improve, stay the same, or perhaps get worse? But as I looked in confusion and uncertainty toward the future,

> In astonishment I could suddenly see
> That in my misery, I had been blind.
> I had a whole garden surrounding me—
> The Present—a place where peace I could find. . . .
>
> So I find myself keeping my garden;
> Sometimes it is hard to tend.
> But I now know that it has always been
> The only garden that is ours in the end.

Then there were the bittersweet occasions, neither utterly discouraging nor purely joyful in their flavor. In the dorm, we had quite a few Scottish exchange students from Edinburgh, and each year they gave a traditional Scottish semiformal dinner dance in honor of the Scottish poet Robert Burns. The evening included men in kilts, a bagpipe concert, and the recital of Burns's poetry. Dinner began with the traditional serving of the haggis.

A group of us had attended the dance each year. I was thrilled that I could make it, and I did enjoy myself. But it was a night of compromises. I had to take the handivan, the university transportation for the handicapped, down to the hotel; I could not walk the distance with my friends. I left early, partly because I was tired. But after dinner, the dancing began, and I did not want to sit at the table by myself or make my friends feel obliged to stay with me. My inability to participate fully could have soured the evening for me, but I reminded myself that at least I was at the party for some of the time. I remembered when I had been at home for the semester, completely physically helpless, unable to join my friends at all. Compared to that time, I was able to do much more. There was another way to think of the night. I could accept it as it was, a present moment, and not judge it in terms of the past. It was my choice whether the night would be bitter or sweet, and I decided in favor of sweetness. That was true for the entire academic year. For those occasions that were bittersweet to me, I rejected bitterness and savored sweetness. I did not want the bitter to become part of me.

I had gone deep into the desert over the past four years, and when I graduated, part of my journey would be coming to an end. I had to decide what road to take next. When I had stood on the mountain of good health, I had planned that I would graduate from Laurel, then fly off to some place new to begin my graduate degree in literature. I had dreamed of California, New York, or maybe New England. Eventually I wanted to settle down somewhere on the east coast, but while I was young and unmarried, I wanted to see all that I could and experience the various ways of life I found in different parts of the country.

I had collected catalogues from universities all over the United States, but when spring arrived, I knew I could not yet leave Philadelphia. At CGH I had found superb physicians; I had an entire medical team caring for me. I knew from past encounters in the medical world that it would not be easy to duplicate such care elsewhere. Also, in Philadelphia, family and friends were nearby in case of emergency.

My parents suggested that I take some time off to rest. They were concerned about the stresses and pressures of graduate school. Since I had become ill, I had been unable to take a full course load, as I would probably have to do in graduate school. But I was determined to go on with my education. Fortunately, I found the perfect solution in Laurel's M.L.A. (Master of Liberal Arts) degree.

In practical terms, the M.L.A. program made sense for me. I would not have to leave Philadelphia. Also, the program was extremely flexible; I did not need to maintain a full-time schedule. I could even receive independent study credit for teaching. I was eligible for federal student loans that would cover tuition. A small amount of the loan would be left over for living expenses.

The M.L.A. program would allow me to fulfill my academic goals. I could continue my research of the relationship between medicine and literature in the way that I wished, by using an interdisciplinary approach. Unlike a Ph.D. program, which would have required a much narrower focus, the M.L.A. encouraged a broader base of study. In my work I would be utilizing the fields of sociology, the history and sociology of science, history, and literature to research the area of literature and medicine. Laurel has one of the best history and sociology of science departments in the country, a resource I intended to make the most of.

Besides, Esther had invited me to teach with her again. I felt a visceral joy when I thought of it. My hands tingled in anticipation of holding a stack of freshly xeroxed syllabi and handing them out to a new class.

Laurel still had a great deal to offer me. After I finished the M.L.A. degree I would then go forth to a different university for my Ph.D. in literature. But I would have had the intellectual freedom to explore the subject of medicine and literature through several fields of study. Hopefully, in a few years, the lupus would be better controlled, and I would no longer need cytoxan treatments. I would not be so tied to CGH. Until then I would still be moving ahead in the general direction I had chosen as I wrote, taught, and performed my research.

Finally, the last week before graduation day arrived, filled with triumphs and festivities. My family attended my induction into Phi Beta Kappa. I was notified that my honors thesis, which had been nominated for three different prizes, had won a national interdisciplinary competition, receiving the Rose Foundation award. "The Weaver" was given an honorable mention in a college poetry competition. And I made the dean's list.

At last it was the day of the College of Arts and Sciences' graduation. I walked across the stage with my class to receive my diploma—a B.A. magna cum laude, with distinction in my major (literature). As he handed me my diploma, the dean stopped me for a moment to congratulate me on the Rose Foundation award. It is a culminating moment etched into my memory.

The next day, Sunday, my parents threw me a graduation party at the Chart House, an elegant restaurant overlooking the river. Family and friends drove in, some from great distances, to share that special day with me. I realized as I looked around the table that, as proud as I was of the awards and honors, they meant far less than the love and friendship surrounding me. I had not traveled through the desert alone; my family and friends had accompanied me and made the journey possible. They were with me now, celebrating my successes and wishing me well as I began down a new road.

There was another in the restaurant with all of us; he had been a guest, though uninvited, throughout the graduation festivities. I saw him, there in the corner, where he had been relegated. I stared into the wolf's yellow eyes, then raised a glass in a silent toast. "You tried, but you did not devour me. You are still here. I have not been able to banish you yet, but I have persevered. I have arrived at this day, which I have made my own, not yours. And I will continue on my way, even with you by my side."

On Monday morning, I went to the graduation ceremony for the entire university. My class paraded down Laurel Walk to the Field, where the event was held. After the ceremony I decided that there was someone I should see. Still dressed in cap and gown, I walked over to Dr. Averapporti's office. I never just dropped in for a visit, but I wanted to thank him. If it were not for his help, I would not have come so far. He had not been able to get me into remission, but with his care, I had been able to remain in school and go on with my life. In that he had given me a great gift, one I had never taken for granted. When I appeared in his office, a huge grin on my face, he came over and gave me a hug. He had never done so before; he is not physically demonstrative. He blushed when I tried to express my gratitude; I knew though, that this day held meaning for us both. And I also knew that, like my family and friends, he would continue to walk with me as I continued on my desert path.

15

A New Path

Summer 1992–Summer 1993

THE SUMMER after graduation I moved into my first apartment, a one-bedroom in a complex located next to the Philadelphia Museum of Art. After living in a dim dorm room on the first floor, I reveled in my sunlit apartment, my aerie on the seventeenth floor. The windows, which stretched the entire length of the apartment, from the dining room, living room to the bedroom, overlooked the Schuylkill River, Boat House Row, and the art museum. I discovered that on July 4, the city shoots off its fireworks in front of the museum. From my windows I had a front-row seat for the display, and laid out below me was the river, bright with the lights of all the small boats whose owners had come for the celebration.

The apartment was furnished with all the love and care my family could give. They transformed that apartment into a home for me. My mom shopped with me on our continuous forays into the stores. I had no idea when I began how much was needed to set up an apartment. Though Dad did not come out with us, his job was essential. He needed to pay the bills! My parents let me take my bedroom furniture and bookshelves from Maryland. The sofa and dinette set were a graduation gift from my grandparents. My brass end table was my aunt's graduation present to me. Bubbe Pearl sent box after box from Florida, filled mostly with kitchenware. Some of it she bought. But what I truly appreciated most were those things that had been hers and her mother's. She sent silver trays and pretty vases. As I write these words, I look up to see my grandmother's Oriental fan spreading itself gracefully over the wall. On my table are silver candlestick holders contributed by Bubbe Leah.

Unpacking was a family enterprise, too. My parents and my brother spent the better part of a week setting everything up for me. I particularly remember my brother painstakingly and patiently putting together an entertainment unit that seemed to have an endless number of parts to which the directions only vaguely and mysteriously referred. Dad uncrated all of my many books and was generally in charge of installing electrical equipment. The kitchen was Mom's territory. She lined the shelves and put everything away. There was a long list of tasks that needed to be done, and my family did not leave me until all was finished.

I have lived here for over four years now, and it is a place of peace and comfort. I gaze around my apartment and take pleasure in it. I suppose that it is not what one would call luxurious. I do not own expensive works of art or antiques. But all around me are objects given to me by friends and family. The people in my life know how much I enjoy going to far-off countries, and though I cannot visit other parts of the world as often as I would like, I travel vicariously through friends who tell me stories of their trips, show me pictures, and always bring me back something for my home. The tiny figurines, four Chinese men who represent the cornerstones of Chinese culture, brought back from Taiwan; the brilliantly clad doll from Brazil; the exquisitely painted soapstone bowls from India; and the nested wooden doll from Russia are only a few of the many gifts I treasure. And though I find these objects aesthetically pleasing, I cherish them not for their beauty, but for the meaning they hold: the strong presence of love and friendship in my life.

I spent the summer acquainting myself with the area surrounding my new home. I must admit that while I was an undergraduate, I, like most of my friends, did not venture away from the university too often. We left campus when we wanted to see movies, go to restaurants and clubs, or shop, but there was much in Philadelphia that we did not explore. So I passed the summer days getting to know the city in which I had lived for the past five years. Sometimes I took the bus into a new part of town and got off at a random spot. From there I walked. I called these excursions my "rambles" about the city. I especially enjoyed the old houses in Society Hill, many of which date from the 1700s and 1800s. I dreamed that someday I would be able to live in such a place. For those houses were endowed with grace and beauty, but also with history—not necessarily the history of prominent people, but the past in all its everyday reality.

I also used my summer vacation to work on my poetry and send it out to literary magazines. I did have some acceptances. I had many rejections, too. But often the rejections proved to be as valuable as the acceptances. Many editors were kind enough to comment on my work, and their suggestions were usually illuminating and helpful. I felt that for the price of postage, I was attending a poetry workshop.

The summer days were pleasant, but I was as always eager to return to school. However, the lupus flared in July, and I worried about having enough strength to begin my graduate studies. I was hospitalized at the end of the month with a severe neurologic attack. As they had in the past, my symptoms mimicked meningitis. I had a terrible headache and sensitivity to light. It was difficult to focus my eyes. All the neurologic and other lupus symptoms I had experienced before also became more pronounced. I was given a spinal tap to rule out infection. The tap was clear; lupus, not meningitis, was the culprit. We raised my steroids and administered another dose of cytoxan. I began physical therapy again. Most of August was a difficult month in terms of my health. I told Dr. Averapporti that his job was to put me back together again in time for school. And when fall arrived, I was feeling better. My symptoms had by no means disappeared, but we had managed to tame them enough for me to begin classes and teaching.

Esther and I again taught our course, "Medicine and Literature: The Physician-Writer," and I was rehired as a WATU Fellow. The basic structure of the course remained the same, though we added and deleted various pieces of literature in each category. More students signed up for the class this time; apparently word had spread. The class had twenty students, the maximum for a seminar. I found teaching to be as exciting as before. Though much of the material did not change, this new group of students made the class completely different. They brought their own perspectives, backgrounds, experiences, and interests; they brought their enthusiasm, too. Their names and faces appear before me now, making me smile. My students.

While teaching, I took my first graduate seminar, an M.L.A. course taught by a historian. The course, "Oral History," was fascinating. For my final project, I managed to tie in my research on medicine and literature. I had long been intrigued by *JAMA's* use of the arts, but did not know how the arts had first become incorporated into *JAMA*. Reading back issues showed me the general increase in the presence of the arts in the journal. But how did this growth come about? In pursuit of an explanation, I went to Chicago, where I interviewed *JAMA's* editor-in-chief, Dr. George Lundberg; Dr. Therese Southgate, the editor responsible, from their inception, for the art covers and cover essays; Charlene Breedlove, the poetry editor; and Roxanne Young, the humanities editor. I collected their oral histories of the story behind the inclusion of the arts in *JAMA*.

I had assumed that the editors had begun with a shared belief in the connection between art and medicine, and from there, had come to a conscious, articulated decision that using art in the journal would benefit *JAMA*'s readers. Today it is true that the editors have highly conceptualized ideas about the relationship between medicine and art. But at the beginning thirty years ago, when the editor-in-chief first decided to put a work of art on the journal cover, it was not because he felt that medicine and art shared some fundamental bond. Far from it; he had merely seen art on corporate magazines and thought the art gave the magazines a classy look. He asked Dr. Southgate, who had no background in art, to write the cover essay. After a great deal of research and anxiety, she finished the essay; though at first, she was quite intimidated by the assignment.

Much to the editors' surprise, the readership responded powerfully and overwhelmingly to the art covers and cover essays. *JAMA* received many letters complimenting and commenting on the new cover and column. Readers even wrote in to complain if Dr. Southgate neglected to write a cover essay. Poetry appeared later, in much the same casual, almost accidental way. And it was also the readers' support of the poetry that made the "Poetry and Medicine" column flourish.

When Dr. Southgate spoke to me about the history of how these art covers and essays had assumed their present form, she concluded, "The art filled a need of some sort . . . that they didn't even know they had . . . The covers touched some nerve. . . . We [the editors] didn't know exactly what need we were filling, but we were responding. The implications and reasons for using the art covers were not thought out at the beginning. But after all, art is a process itself. *JAMA* reflected this in the way in which [the art covers] evolved, too." In the history of how art came to be such an integral part of *JAMA*, I found further confirmation of an inherent relationship between the arts and medicine.

I flew back from Chicago excited by all that I had learned. I could not wait to share my experiences with Esther and my students. But, as had been true in the past, the satisfaction I derived from my work did not protect me against the ravages of the disease. I continued to ride the roller coaster of symptoms and treatments. I still underwent cytoxan treatments every month; over time, we had gradually raised the dosage. I know that Dr.

Averapporti wrote out each cytoxan order with dread, afraid of the accumulated harm he might be doing to my body. But we both feared the disease more. With each cytoxan infusion, Dr. Averapporti and I hoped that this would be the one that would bring sustained relief. We could then wean me away from the cytoxan and reduce my steroid dosage. Dr. Averapporti and I desperately wanted to decrease my steroids. I was gaining more weight and filling with fluid. Dr. Averapporti was concerned, too, about my bones, because with long-term use steroids can cause osteoporosis. My disease quieted down after each cytoxan dose, but after a few weeks, the disease became active once more.

In the first week of December, I went to the emergency room. The involuntary movements, jerking, twitching, trembling, and shaking had become severe, and I was having multiple attacks each day. My other symptoms, particularly the neurologic ones, were worse as well. The neurology resident in the ER wanted to hospitalize me, though I was not enthusiastic about this. Once the involuntary movements subsided, I was ready to go home. But he convinced me to stay.

I was fortunate that he did so. The next day, the neurology team, including the resident who had seen me the previous day, came in to visit my roommate. But while they were in the middle of examining her, I began to spasm again. My limbs stiffened, then twitched and jerked. My eyelids fluttered rapidly. The muscles in my face were also jumping. As this was happening, the resident from the night before just happened to look over at me. He interrupted the attending physician, Dr. Fields, and motioned toward me. The team hurried over.

As Dr. Fields examined me, he carefully explained his findings to the residents, the medical students, and to me. His first concern was to ascertain whether or not I was aware of my surroundings and oriented in terms of time and place. It was hard for me to respond, though I did manage. I understood him and knew what I wanted to say, but the muscles in my jaw were rigid and tight. The loss of motor control in my mouth made speaking difficult. Dr. Fields asked me where I would most like to be at that moment. I did not have to think long. "In the Caribbean!" I answered. The entire neurology team laughed at that. Now that Dr. Fields was sure that I was alert and conscious, he tested all of my reflexes, from my ankles to my eyes. After he was done, he pronounced, "Her reflexes are all extremely brisk. She has myoclonus."

Myoclonus can be defined as sudden, brief, shocklike involuntary movements caused by muscle contractors or inhibitors. Myoclonus can originate anywhere in the central nervous system—from the cortex, the brain stem, or the spinal cord. If it comes from the cortex, which is the higher part of the brain, myoclonus can be a form of seizure. Dr. Fields ordered an EEG to determine whether I was experiencing seizures or myoclonus. The EEG was negative, and he decided that the source of the myoclonus was not the brain. Much to my relief, I was not having seizures. The MRI of my brain was also negative, though I knew that the MRI does not conclusively rule out brain involvement in lupus. It was assumed that the myoclonus was coming from inflammation in my spinal cord.

I was given an anti-spasticity drug, baclofen, which is also used to treat myoclonus. The drug took immediate effect, particularly in my hands. I noticed that my hands were relaxing, becoming far less rigid and stiff. I was kept in the hospital for just a few days. On the last day I spoke with Dr. Fields. I had been followed by a CGH neurologist who had recently left, and I needed a replacement. I liked this doctor. He had a no-nonsense air about him, but his blue eyes were kind and his hands gentle. I appreciated his wry sense of humor. I felt an immediate rapport with him. Most important, he had been able to make sense out of what was happening and prescribe an effective treatment quickly.

I said, "Dr. Fields, there is something I want to ask you. I was really impressed with the way you've been handling my care these past few days. Would you be my neurologist?" "It would be my pleasure," he said. He held out his hand, and I offered my own. We shook hands as if we had just agreed on an important contract. Despite the seriousness of his gesture, he had a twinkle and a smile in his eyes. In that brief exchange I felt reassured. Here was another person, compassionate and knowledgeable, who would join me in my battles with the wolf. Someone I could depend upon and trust.

Then it was the end of the term. But I did not have the strength to finish my work on time, and I had to take an incomplete in my oral history seminar. I spent the first two weeks of the break writing my final paper for that course, then decided to visit my grandparents in Florida. I thought a little bit of rest, relaxation, and being absolutely spoiled would be a pleasant way to end my vacation.

Unfortunately, I was not feeling well during the trip. But one particularly frightening episode took place toward the end of my four-day weekend. This attack differed from my usual myoclonic attacks. I became very sleepy, and my head was so heavy, a leaden weight. My eyes were sensitive to the light. My grandparents were on their way out to do a bit of shopping.

They came over to me before they left, and my grandmother said later that my speech was slurred, my eyes half-closed and glassy. They made me lie down. I mumbled that I was just tired. After they left the house, the jerking began. I remember my body going rigid and then spasming once; after that, nothingness. When I awoke, I was cold, weak, and slightly disoriented.

This was not the first such episode. Over the past few weeks, I had experienced milder but similar attacks. I had told no one; I did not want to admit that my myoclonic attacks were becoming more severe. After the episode in Florida, I realized that I could no longer ignore what was happening. When I returned to school, I called my rheumatologist and my neurologist. I had three questions about these latest episodes. Was I now suffering from seizures? If so, what should we do? Were these episodes dangerous?

Dr. Fields concluded that my attacks were a combination of seizures and myoclonus, but he strongly felt that the answer did not lie in doping me with neurologic drugs. The primary goal must be to control the lupus and prevent further damage to my nervous system. Neurologic drugs addressed only the symptoms, not the root cause, which was my overactive immune system. My two basic choices for treating the lupus were to stay on the present cytoxan regimen or to alternate the cytoxan with pulse steroid infusions. The thought of using high dose steroid treatments on a regular basis made me cringe. The likelihood of my suffering the many steroid-related side effects would dramatically increase with frequent high dose exposure. So I chose to continue the cytoxan without the pulse steroids. At least I would only risk the toxicity of the one treatment, not two.

I was deeply frightened by the seizures, not only by the events themselves, but also by all they implied. It was then that I confronted what I could not face before. The beast was no longer content with just my spinal cord; the wolf was now gnawing on my brain. For the past two years, Dr. Averapporti had wondered whether I had what was then called "lupus cerebritis" (brain inflammation caused by lupus). But I did not have a definitive diagnosis until now. So, up until this time, I chose not to believe. But now the possibility was reality. My brain was diseased.

The phrase "brain disease" flew about my mind like an angry wasp, stinging, drawing blood each time it settled. How I wished it were my liver, kidneys, or lungs under assault. Anything but my brain. My brain defined my identity in a way that no other organ did. My brain housed my intellect, personality, and memories, all that I most treasured about myself. I could bear the accumulated loss of my physical abilities, because I made the distinction between myself and my ill body; my body was diseased, but *I* was well.

But if my brain, that which sustained and created the *I* of Melissa, was diseased, then *I* was diseased. When lupus involves the brain, it commonly causes cognitive and psychiatric problems. What if I lost the powers of my intellect? My view of life and the world? My way of interacting and connecting with others? I would suffer the ultimate loss. I would lose myself. And I would not possess the ability to fight the disease as I had before, because my weapons came from my brain, the organ that allowed me to think, feel, act, and choose.

But, as I had done in the past, I sank my fear and grief like a stone into a lake I hid deep within me. I tried to ignore the seizures and all that they signified to me. The seizures would come, and when they were over, I pushed the memory of them back into the furthest recesses of my mind. I did not forget or repress the memory; I just refused to think of it. For a long time I would not even say the word "seizure," even in my mind, as if saying it would make it more real, confirm it in some way. Instead, I called the seizures "episodes." Since I had become ill, I had always read voraciously about my disease, for knowledge meant power and control. But I did not pick up a single book or article about epilepsy. I would not think of myself as an epileptic.

Then, a few weeks after speaking with Dr. Fields, I was walking in the city and saw an ambulance parked in the street. A small crowd had gathered. They were staring at a man having a seizure. Stripped of all dignity and control, the man jerked and convulsed on the sidewalk. But the most awful thing of all, from my perspective, was the gaze of the crowd, who watched, unable to tear themselves away. It was both fascination and disgust I saw on their faces, as if they were watching a kind of live horror movie. I walked away as fast as I could go. But I could not outwalk the realization that even though I was part of the crowd today, at any time, I could become the man on the sidewalk—helpless, humiliated.

I returned to my apartment. I wanted to hide away in my aerie and never go back down. My brain was damaged, and now I had seizures and violent myoclonic attacks during which I was completely, physically helpless. And who knew what other havoc the lupus could wreak in my brain?

But then that strong, truthful inner voice on which I have always relied said, "You don't have to be powerless when you're not having a seizure. That's your choice." I paused, joy filling me. That voice, which came from the most basic part of myself, was with me; *I* was still here. At least for the moment, my power to think and reason, as well as my fierce desire to continue on with my life, were intact. Would it remain so? I did not know what the future held for me and the *I* of me. But I realized that *I* could put myself in a jail, creating prison bars out of what might be, destroying myself as certainly as the lupus could by further inflaming by brain. Or *I* could choose to keep the *I* in me alive and free, for as long as I possibly could. Maybe that would even be for the rest of my life. I could not know. And there lay hope and fear.

The next day I was asked if I wanted to go with a group of friends to the movies. I hesitated a moment. What if I had a seizure while I was with them? Then I said, "Yes." I chose freedom.

I stayed faithful to that decision; I never became a recluse. I went my way about the city and the campus, continuing on with my usual routine. I never turned down an invitation, even to travel, out of fear that I might have a seizure. But when I look back to that time when the seizures were a new presence in my life, I realize that my freedom was only partial. For at the beginning, I went to great lengths to hide the seizures from everyone— my family, my friends, my colleagues, even my health-care professionals.

Whenever I felt an attack coming on, my first instinct was to hide. I became adept at covering, appearing normal, during those first ten or fifteen minutes before a seizure when I began to receive the warning signs of lethargy, slurred speech, dizziness, loss of balance, headache, nausea, and blurred vision. At the first hint of trouble, before my problems became overwhelmingly obvious, I would make my escape. If someone noticed I was unwell, I would shrug and say, "Oh, yes, I think I'm coming down with the flu," or "I've been working so hard, I'm just exhausted." All over campus I had places I could tuck myself away until the seizure was over. I learned that if I were in a department store, a dressing room offered a safe haven.

Why did I act this way? There is no simple explanation. But I know that this latest terrifying violation of my body, my self, made me grieve again, deeply. And when we mourn, we deny. I reverted to behaving the way I used to do after I was first diagnosed with the illness. If no one else saw the seizures, I could pretend they were not happening, or at least I could more easily ignore them. I was protecting myself. And others as well. For even though the rational, intellectual part of me knew that seizures should not be viewed differently from any of my other symptoms, so powerful is the stigma of epilepsy, I could not help but feel a lingering sense of shame and embarrassment about the seizures. If I felt this way, how would other people react, especially my friends and colleagues? Would I lose them if they saw me having a seizure?

Anger, too, as well as denial, was part of the grief process, part of coming to terms with the seizures. One memory comes to me. I was in my apartment. I felt the seizure begin, the unnatural drowsiness and lethargy stealing over me. As I lay on my couch, which was soft powder blue with a pastel floral pattern, it was as if I were transported to my inner garden that the wolf had so ruthlessly plundered. I saw him there, the beast with his mangy gray pelt, sharp claws, and vicious teeth.

He became aware of my presence. Our eyes locked. With all the power born of my outrage at the trampled garden, I shouted, "NO! GET OUT!" I felt this piercing scream might have shattered glass if it could have been uttered out loud. The wolf, in his surprise, seemed to hesitate a moment. For a split second I thought that the seizure would stop. But then the tingling began in my feet, and my legs tightened, stiffened. My cries became lost in gathering winds of that electric storm which silences speech and cancels being. As my jaw clamped shut, I felt my whole body convulse in one hard jerk—then nothingness. Several hours later, I pulled myself slowly, sluggishly toward the waking world, which was unfamiliar and confusing when I arrived. Time and place were jumbled. Eventually I solved these puzzles and lurched to my feet.

The number, type, and severity of the seizures I experienced each day and each week varied. I will estimate that on a really bad day, I had three or four seizures similar to the one I had in Florida with my grandparents, and in a rough week, I had at least one seizure or severe myoclonic attack every day. I always became ill before each seizure; lost consciousness during, and felt sleepy, woozy, and disoriented after. So a really bad day meant that I was basically in some part of the seizure stage all day long. The absolute physical and mental exhaustion after such a string of seizures was ravaging and lasted for at least a day or two, even if those next few days were seizure-free.

But usually the seizures were smaller events that occurred more often, though these were enough to slow me down, make me feel drained and less alert. I once asked Dr. Averapporti why this was so. Why did a seizure that might be over in only a few minutes make me feel tired and my mind dulled? He said to think of it this way: it is as if your brain is a computer that has been zapped by an electrical storm, first a power surge and then a power outage. When you reboot your machine, it takes a little while for all the programs to run smoothly again. As these interruptions in power continue to take place, it strains your brain to keep stopping and starting improperly.

To help deal with the stress of the increasing disease activity, I had continued to go to lupus support group meetings. But the meetings were less comforting than they had been in the past. Part of that was my own reluctance to discuss the worst of my lupus symptoms. I felt protective of the other people in the group. I did not want them to hear about my complicated neurologic involvement and worry that they would experience the same symptoms or require similar treatments. But in keeping silent, I only felt more isolated.

Then one night early in the spring semester, I attended a meeting that was to be my last. On my left was a mother who had lost her daughter, a young woman my age, to lupus. On my right were a mother and daughter whose entire family had been devastated by lupus. Several years before, the father and son had died of lupus nephritis. The daughter, Yvonne, was critically ill from her disease. She had a blood disorder caused by the lupus; her physicians had told her that even a cut could kill her. They would not be able to stop the bleeding. Yvonne said in a bleak, hopeless voice, "It's like living on the edge of a cliff, knowing you could be pushed off any moment." Yvonne had an older sister who also had lupus; the sister was too sick to attend the meeting. Yvonne's mother was the only family member free of the disease, but she was forced to stand by, utterly helpless, as her family suffered and died from lupus.

What could I say? What could I do to ease the pain and anguish of the mother whose daughter had died or Yvonne and her mother? I felt powerless to be of any service to them, except to listen and bear witness to their sorrow. Not only could I not help these people, but their accounts made real to me the possibility of dying of this disease. Before, I had worried about the ways in which the disease could affect my quality of life, but I had not seriously thought that I could die from lupus. Disability, not death, concerned me. But that meeting had been haunted with the specter of death, and I wanted no part of it. I never went back again.

For weeks after that meeting, I was disturbed by all that I had heard and felt. I remember talking on the telephone to a friend of mine from my undergraduate days. She joked, "Oh, I can picture all of us when we're ninety years old. We'll have outlived our husbands and you, me, Mary, and Teresa will be sitting on rocking chairs in the old-age home, gossiping just like we do now." I laughed, but fleetingly, the thought passed through my mind, "Will I live that long? Will I die of this disease before I reach old age?"

However, as time passed, the fears blessedly receded. Yvonne had told the group that it seemed as if she lived at the edge of a cliff. But all of us, as mortal, fragile human beings, live precariously, with no absolute security or guarantees. We are all cliff-edge dwellers. I could become paralyzed by fright as I stared down the sheer drop to the unknown blackness below. Or I could dance with joy on the cliff's edge, embracing the night and day, stars and sun. I chose to dance. I turned away from thoughts of death and toward the things I had always found reassuring and sustaining—my relationships with others and my work. My satisfaction in my school life never dimmed; in a world made chaotic by illness, it was my center that always held.

Odd though it might seem, it took me much longer to sort through my feelings about the seizures than it did to deal with my fear of dying from the disease. The frightening specter of death appeared relatively quickly, directly, and I was able to deal with it in the way that it had come. Not so with the seizures. The seizures came into my life in a slow, sneaky way, carrying a load of baggage with them. They packed social stigma and the personal meaning of brain disease in their heavy luggage. I needed a lot of time to get used to the seizures, the events themselves and all their attached baggage. I could not just say to myself, "Accept seizures as a part of your life and be comfortable that others will too." The mind will decide to accept, but the heart will still mourn.

I did eventually stop hiding the seizures from my health-care professionals, family, friends, and close colleagues—at least most of the time. I did not lose my friends and colleagues, as I had so worried I might. Veterans of my illness, they only wanted to know what they needed to do if I should have a seizure. My friends continued to invite me on every trip, to every event. My seizures never changed how they thought of me. Yet my first reaction when I felt a seizure come on continued to be a feeling of embarrassment and an urge to take cover, even if I did not always act on them. For me, this was as completely as I accepted the seizures.

But my life did not stop while I was struggling to reach this semi-acceptance of the seizures, a gradual process that took place over several years. I continued to walk the path I had chosen for myself, and in that, I remained free. I pursued my education with the same enthusiasm as always, and in the spring semester of 1993, it was a literary theory course that especially occupied my mind.

The class, "English Literary Criticism: From Wordsworth to T. S. Eliot," was a small graduate seminar with only six or seven students. The professor, Dr. Roberts, was a phenomenal teacher, the scope and depth of whose knowledge was enormous. He brought history, current events, and art to our discussions of literature, and he was extremely approachable and interested in his students. In him I found another guide, friend, and mentor.

I became very involved in writing my term paper, "A Mirror to This Modernity: William Carlos Williams and William Wordsworth," for Professor Roberts's class. Though Williams consciously and emphatically breaks from the poetic traditions of his Romantic forefathers, including Wordsworth, it seems to me that Williams and Wordsworth are still profoundly linked. Williams finds his poetry in the immediate, brutal, poverty-stricken world of the people in Paterson, New Jersey. The wellspring of Wordsworth's poetry is in the "low and rustic" life and people of the countryside, a group that the literate society of his time generally viewed as devoid of importance, meaning, and even humanity. Both poets value common people and their experiences. Wordsworth's and Williams's sources yield very different poetry and literary innovations. But each writer creates his poetry in the firm belief that poetry can act as a protective and uniting force in the wounded, fragmented, modern world.

Through this research into the relationship between Williams and Wordsworth, I was continuing to affirm and assert my conviction that literature may powerfully serve as a living, healing force in the everyday world of modern life. I discovered my literary heroes and models in writers like Williams and Wordsworth who found a vital connection between immediate experience and writing.

That spring term was intellectually exciting, but the disease kept its fierce grip on me. Early in the semester, I began to experience strange visual distortions. At first they were subtle, and I told myself that I was just worn out by my schedule. I argued with myself that the misperceptions were not that abnormal, even as part of me wondered if I were just finally losing my mind. But then the episodes became more pronounced. I was reversing letters. Sometimes letters would drop out of a word. The oddest incident occurred as I was walking down my hallway toward my bathroom. To the left was the door to my bedroom. I stopped by my bedroom door, puzzled and confused by what I was seeing. I could not see the door, just an expanse of whiteness without borders or definition. I thought perhaps the door was open and I was looking out the window into dense fog, though that explanation did not seem quite right. I moved forward to investigate and ran into the door. Once I made physical contact with the door, I realized what I had been seeing. But the incident left me shaken.

I decided that I could no longer keep these visual distortions to myself, but I did not have the courage to go directly to my doctor. First, I consulted my mother. I knew that some of the people she tutored had trouble reading because they reversed letters. I wondered if my symptoms would sound familiar to her. I explained what had been happening, and she said that many of her students had visual perceptual problems. She advised me to call Dr. Averapporti; these visual distortions were significant, and I should not ignore them. Dr. Averapporti was very concerned about these problems with my visual perception. He felt that I was experiencing periodic episodes during which my brain did not get enough oxygen; the oxygen deprivation was causing these distortions.

I also continued to have seizures. Physical exertion seemed to bring them on. I kept having attacks while I was in physical therapy. In the middle of February I landed in the emergency room because of the seizures. For months the nurses in the SPU had seen the seizures and the myoclonus. At the beginning of March, while I was receiving a cytoxan treatment in the SPU, I went into a seizure again. I was unresponsive for an extended period of time. Karen, the nurse who was caring for me, became extremely worried—and angry. She called my rheumatologist and my neurologist and demanded that they come down to the SPU and see for themselves what was happening. And she wanted me to be treated for the seizures. NOW. The seizures had gone on long enough, in her opinion; I needed some relief.

Dr. Averapporti and Dr. Fields did visit me in the SPU that day. They decided to prescribe Dilantin, a common anticonvulsant. Because of my sensitivity to drugs, the doctors began with a small dosage, then gradually increased it. To be effective, Dilantin must reach a blood level that falls within a therapeutic range, and it took us several months to build up to that level. Meanwhile, the lupus remained out of control. At the end of May I was hospitalized, given my cytoxan treatment, and then discharged.

At the beginning of that summer, my parents moved to Valley Forge, a suburb of Philadelphia. They had told me about the move a few months earlier, when they came into the city for the Passover holiday. During the dinner my mom seemed jumpy and anxious. I asked her several times if something was the matter, but she said that everything was fine. After the meal at my grandmother's, my mother, accompanied by my aunt and grandmother, drove me back to my apartment. They insisted on coming up with me, though I kept dropping hints that I was exhausted and would rather continue our visit the next day. My mother, grandmother, and aunt sat down on the couch. My mother explained nervously, "Melissa, I wanted to talk to you about something. Your father and I decided to move up here to Philadelphia. We can't stay in the Maryland house; we can't afford it anymore. You know your father has had troubles with the business. We have to move anyway, and it would make it a lot easier on us to be nearer to you.

I wouldn't have to drive such a long distance for your treatments. And I worry about you. I hate being so far away. I know you're going to be upset, but this is what we're going to do." She looked at me, ready for battle. She knew I cherished my independence, and she was sure that I would consider their moving to Philadelphia a threat. She had even brought my grandmother and aunt with her for moral support.

But perhaps for the first time in our lives, I took my mother completely by surprise. Without missing a beat, I answered, "Mom, I'm not upset about your coming to Philadelphia. If that's what you want to do, then that's fine with me. But when you move to Philadelphia, you and Dad can't center your life around me. That wouldn't be healthy for any of us. You both have to make your own life here. After all, when I finish with the M.L.A. program, I'll probably leave the city to go to another graduate school. And you two can't follow me around the country. But as long as we understand each other, I'm glad you'll be here. Did you expect that I would take a map, draw a large circle around Philadelphia, and say you couldn't move within a certain number of miles from me?" My mother was flabbergasted, rendered utterly speechless by my calm acquiescence to the move.

My parents have remained in the suburban Philadelphia area since then, and it has worked out well for all of us. My father brought his full-time business from Maryland to Philadelphia. He still mainly works from home, writing mathematics and computer science textbooks as well as developing computer software. About ten years before, he had resigned his position as tenured professor at the University of Maryland so that he could devote himself completely to his company. He never regretted that decision, but he missed working with students. When he moved back to Philly, my father began teaching again on a class-by-class basis at one of the many nearby universities.

Mom and I have benefited from the move. Closing the miles between us makes her feel more secure, more peaceful. And I must admit that my parents' proximity has made my own life easier. I try not to become overly dependent, but when I am really not feeling well, my parents are able to help me. My mom occasionally stocks my kitchen with groceries when I am too tired to shop. One time she even went with me to the library. I did a library search on the computer, then sent her to gather the materials and make the photocopies. This saved me a lot of energy. Many times I go to my parents' house to rest, recuperate, and enjoy some animal therapy, administered by my parents' four cats and two dogs.

I realize how far my parents and I have traveled since those early days of my illness. Today, I accept their help; I do not turn them away. For they do not shelter their "sick child" from the world; they give practical support in an attempt to enable me to do all I can and be as independent as possible. We have finally formed a healing circle of giving and receiving help in which we all recognize each other's needs. When the lupus flares, creating new needs for all of us, the circle can be broken. But we are able to reconnect the circle, encompassing whatever changes have come to pass.

Throughout the summer, the disease activity was unrelenting. Seizures brought me to the emergency room at the beginning of June; and in both July and August, I was hospitalized for lupus flares. Then, at the end of the summer, the seizures subsided. The Dilantin had finally built up to a therapeutic level in my bloodstream. Unfortunately, at this blood level, the side effects of the drug became intolerable. The Dilantin-induced vertigo was so intense that I could not even walk around my apartment. I was given medication for the vertigo, but the drug only made me extremely nauseous. I was taken off the Dilantin, and the seizures returned.

But at the end of August I gathered what little physical strength I possessed to attend a college friend's wedding in Atlanta. I traveled with a few other friends from college. We made a vacation out of our time in Atlanta, renting a car and touring the city and its outskirts. The wedding was a traditional southern affair, conservative and sedate, and very different from the rather boisterous Jewish weddings to which I was accustomed. As I watched my friend standing beside his bride, tears in his eyes as he recited his wedding vows, I felt overwhelmingly grateful that I could be there that day to share in this event. Those few days were a celebration and a respite, a brief hiatus from illness, doctors, and hospitals. But all too soon, it was time to return home.

16

Another Fork in the Road

Fall 1993–Spring 1995

S UMMER BECAME fall, and it was time for the new academic year. But by now the lupus, especially the neurologic manifestations, had been flaring out of control for months. My vision was affected in a number of ways. I was having problems with depth perception, peripheral vision, and cognitive visual perception. The difficulties with my eyes complicated another lupus symptom—my poor balance. Because of my sensory losses in the lower half of my body, it was difficult to maintain my balance, but I had compensated by using my sight. Now I could not depend on my eyes, and my balance became more precarious. It was also hard for me to read. In part this was because I had trouble focusing my eyes, but I also misperceived letters. Objects frequently lost their identity and turned into puzzling oddities. There were episodes when the scenery fell apart, the landscape turning into jumbled and fragmented pieces.

The most terrifying aspect of the visual distortions was my increasing inability to recognize people. Late in the spring semester, I met a woman on three distinct occasions. First, we sat across from each other while riding the apartment shuttle. She taught at the university, and we spoke of her experiences in the classroom. Next we stood near one another while we picked out produce in the apartment building's commissary. Her little girl accompanied her. This time the woman and I talked about the quality of the fruit and commiserated over the high prices. I never realized that she was the same woman I had met earlier on the bus.

On the third encounter, she mentioned her class at the university. Later in the conversation, she asked if I would like to come grocery shopping at a larger supermarket where the prices would be cheaper. The conversation, not the face, formed the connection, and I realized that the professor from the bus, the mother in the commissary, and the woman to whom I was now speaking were the same individual.

I experienced other episodes in which the distortions were not visual but auditory. The conversation to which I had been listening would suddenly become garbled, as if the person had begun speaking a language which I did not know. After a minute or two, I would twitch, and I could then understand what was being said. I experienced some seizures in which I just disappeared for a few minutes. When I became aware again, I would realize that time had passed. For example, perhaps the radio had been playing a particular song, but when I came back to myself, a new song was on.

Most horrific of all were the difficulties I was having with my thinking. Words had always been mine to command. Yet my illness was stealing them away. For months I refused to admit the burglary of my expression. But so often now, when I tried to write, my thoughts and ideas were shrouded in a fog I struggled to penetrate. An idea would hover in my mind, and I would rush to capture it in words, but both words and idea would elude me, fade away. During the spring and summer, I had short periods when the mists cleared, and then I worked with fierce concentration, rushing to record my thoughts before they were lost to me. This is how I continued with my studies.

By fall it had been months since I had written a poem. When I tried to write poetry, the image around which I intended to build the piece was etched in my mind, the snapshot given substance and color by the emotions and thoughts associated with it. But as I tried to translate the vivid technicolor into the music of poetry, I knew that the flat, jangling, and discordant phrases bore no, or little, relation to what was in my mind.

Other episodes of confusion went far beyond the visual and auditory distortions and terrified me more than even my decreasing ability to write. One day in early September I was restlessly prowling my apartment, unable to study, fighting lethargy, pain, and self-pity. I looked out my window to the sunny day, unusually cool and crisp for that time of year, and decided to go out for a bit to the nearby record store, where I could buy what my Bubbe Pearl calls a "perky." Maybe I could lose my self-pity, if not my medical problems, in the snap of the fall breeze, letting that ugly emotion fall away from me like curled brown leaves from autumn trees.

I boarded the apartment shuttle. I would get off at its midway point, fifteen minutes later, and walk one block to the store. As I sat on the bus, my fatigue grew worse, and a headache began to build. Still, I got off the bus. Somehow, in my now increasingly muddled mind, reaching the store had assumed the importance of finding the Holy Grail. If I made it, then I proved to myself, and the wolf, that I could not be beaten. I would not succumb to the illness or self-pity.

As I stood on a street corner usually as familiar to me as the rooms of my own apartment, lethargy overwhelmed me, and the headache reached a pounding crescendo. I became completely disoriented. I could see everything around me—people rushing by, buildings, traffic. I could even read the street signs, but the numbers and names meant nothing to me. I did not know how to get to the record store or even how to return home. When I reached into my mind, I was able to find some words and ideas, but I could not connect them together in a coherent way. So I could not even ask for help, because I did not know how to explain my problem. I began to panic. I no longer cared about the record store. I just wanted to go home, where I would be safe. But how? As the people passed by me, I felt completely alone. And mute. And trapped.

Out of the chaos of my mind, I registered that a taxi was parked near me. I knew that this was a way of escape. I stumbled into the cab. When the driver asked, "Where to, miss?" I could not answer, having forgotten my own address. But I drew upon the little clarity of mind I had left to search my purse. I found my appointment book, in which I had written my address on the first page. I showed it to the driver.

In this way I managed to reach my apartment. It was late afternoon, and I fell onto the couch, sleeping there through the night. When I awoke, the headache and the overwhelming lethargy were gone. Most important, my mind had returned to some semblance of order, at least compared to my massive confusion of the day before.

By the early fall, I was experiencing few periods of clarity. The dense fog thickened and thinned. It left me enough awareness to know and mourn all the power of mind that I had lost, yet I remained powerless to do anything about it, even to speak of it to another through my writing and receive the healing gift of understanding. By this time, writing was an impossibility; my conduit of words had finally been severed.

At the beginning of September, I went to the eye doctor's office for my yearly checkup to make sure that the Plaquenil was not damaging my retinas. Feverish, my joints swollen, hot, and aching, my head pounding, I dragged myself to the office. I sat in the waiting room, a crowded little box with no windows. A half hour became forty-five minutes, then an hour. Every ten or fifteen minutes, my limbs would stiffen and jerk in brief myoclonic spasms.

The longer I waited, the more I felt that the room was becoming smaller, its walls pressing closer together. With every minute, my anger grew. I thought of the bright summer day outside the hospital. *That* was where I should be. Outside, feeling the warmth of the sun on my face. Free. I could not wait in one more doctor's office, nor spend one more second in illness's domain. No more. Usually polite to the extreme, and reconciled to waiting for my medical appointments, I glared at every person passing by— other patients, technicians, secretaries, and most of all, the doctors who were keeping me hostage here. I called out to a secretary who walked by me, "When is the doctor going to see me? If he doesn't call me in the next five minutes, I'm leaving. This is ridiculous." Surprised at my tone and attitude, she scurried off to ask the doctor when he would be ready for me. I was known in this office as "Smiley" and "Miss Sunshine." But there was nothing cheery about me that day. When the doctor finally ushered me into his office two hours after my appointment time, he apologized for the wait. I did not even let him finish. I snapped, "Let's just get this over with. I'm in a hurry."

I returned home in a foul mood. Furious, upset, frightened, soul-weary from everything that had been happening over the past months, I turned to all that had helped ease my grief in the past. I longed to take a walk by the river. The sun would be warm against my back as I watched the crew boats, our city river swans, glide elegantly over the glinting blue surface. I would pet the dogs being walked and pass a few moments of friendly conversation with their owners. "What kind of dog is this? A black lab? My mom has samoyeds. I grew up with dogs." And I would feel connected again to the mundane, everyday world outside myself and my illness. But I did not have the strength to go. I looked toward the phone, thinking of calling a friend or a family member. Yet that was not open to me either. I was too physically drained to maintain a conversation. Besides, my friends and family, in all their healthy normalcy, seemed far removed from me, and today the distance was too great to bridge. I knew that I did not have the power of mind to write; the words were hidden in the fog. But I hoped that I could borrow other people's words until my own were returned to me. I picked up a book of William Carlos Williams's poetry and settled on the couch. My hands were shaking so badly that I could scarcely turn the pages or hold the book. I eventually found my favorite poem for which I was searching. But I could not read it. My eyes could not make sense of it. With a keening cry, I hurled the book at the wall. At least that was my intent, though in my weakened condition, I did not throw the book very hard. Still, it hit the nearby wall and fell to the floor with a small thud, landing cover up, the pages beneath crumpled, the spine cracked, a broken body with torn cream flesh.

I went into my room and crawled into bed. Lying curled on my side, I was devoured by a grief that left me nothing, not even the release of tears. In its wake, my mind became blank, empty and dark, as if a twister had swept across it. I do not know how long I lay like this, but gradually there arose a cry out of my black quiet, a wordless expression of the deepest need. It did not go unheeded. For it was then that the Light came to me, every part of me, filling the emptiness, transforming the darkness. The Light grew ever stronger, until it assumed an unspeakably powerful, beneficent radiance. Not a word had been uttered during these moments, for I did not experience the Light in words, only in images and emotions beyond language. But I knew I was in the presence of the Source who had created the world and lived in its core. Gradually the Light faded, leaving me, but not alone. Never again alone. For I had been given a revelation and a promise of its presence, in the world, in my life. I began to drift, my grief eased, borne to a healing sleep on hands made of Light.

I awoke the next day. My illness was not gone from me by any means, but the worst of my anguish had passed. I went about my daily round. I did not analyze what had happened the day before. The Light was something that I *knew* in a way that I did not *know* anything else. It had become a part of me, like the blood running through my veins, and did not need to be assessed by my intellect.

Now that I do use my reasoning powers in looking at my experience of the Light, part of me wonders, for just an instant, did this come out of my own desperate need? Am I maker of the Light? Creator of the Creator? Or even more terrible to contemplate, was my experience of the Light only the result of a seizure, a product of my disease? There are some physicians who think Joan of Arc was an epileptic who, unaware of her disease, believed that her seizures were visions sent by God. I have no definitive answers for these questions. I only know that the Light is real, within me and without. I cannot prove it. But that is the essence of faith. A certainty in the unknowable.

As I think about it now, I realize that I had at last found a faith I could call my own—one as solid and enduring as the Christianity of Teresa and Kim. Mine had no name, no church, no identifiable followers, yet I am united with all who believe that a Maker built this world and fashioned its core out of grace, beauty, and meaning. A Maker who watches over his creation with involved compassion.

I never did talk of my newfound faith to anyone. It felt too private, as if to speak of it would be like shedding all my clothes and running naked through the streets. I kept it a secret part of me until the writing of this book. I have entrusted this to you because I owe you the truth of my life and my journey as I know it. And my gaining knowledge of the Light is an essential part of my story. It is only now that I understand that. I had been searching for the Light since my childhood, before I became ill. Would I have found my way to my faith, even if the wolf had not come to me? Is this a gift of the beast? I will never know, of course. But I sense that somehow, even if my life had gone another direction, through the valley and not the desert, I would have learned of the Light.

It is with my faith that I have traveled on. My faith does not keep the wolf from me or spare me from grieving each time the beast attacks. But the blackness of mourning no longer touches the deepest part of me, for that part is filled with indestructible Light. Beyond the grief lies the certainty my faith gives me that I am not alone, in the most fundamental sense, and that life has meaning, beauty, and possibility even in the midst of suffering and loss. In this certainty I find strength.

Despite the disease's continual onslaught, this sense of security stayed with me and sustained me. I brought it with me to the hospital when, at the end of September, I was admitted to CGH for two weeks. At the very beginning of my stay, before any real testing was conducted, I had a severe myoclonic attack. A nurse called in a member of the house staff, and he said, "Oh, that's just myoclonus, not a seizure. Give her some oxygen. That usually helps myoclonus." I was placed on oxygen, and I immediately responded. The myoclonus ceased, and I became more aware and alert.

Later the neurologists came in to see me. They wanted to know why I was receiving oxygen. I explained that an intern or resident, I was not sure which, had ordered it, and it had stopped a myoclonic attack. They were amazed and intrigued by the role that oxygen was playing. During that time, many specialists came in to see me—neurologists, neuro-ophthalmologists, neurologists who specialized in cognition, rheumatologists, and pulmonary specialists. They were all utterly fascinated by my symptoms and the relief the oxygen was giving me. I had become what is known as an "interesting case."

Through an MRI with an oxygenation study, a xenon blood flow test, and a SPECT scan, the neurologists determined that my brain, specifically my visual cortex, was not receiving enough oxygen. The physicians were greatly excited by their findings. The SPECT scan was an experimental test favored by the rheumatologists; the xenon blood flow was an experimental study developed and preferred by the CGH neurologists. Each side argued for the superiority of its particular test. In my case, both tests correlated directly with my symptoms, and both the neurologists and the rheumatologists saw the results as validating their method of study.

I appreciated their dedication and enthusiasm, but I was beginning to feel consumed by it all.

As I lie under the white blankets,
they come to me
white robed men and women
flooding my hospital room,
waves of white washing into white;
soon I become lost
in relentless white tides.

They peer deep into my eyes
through the blackness of pupil
then wheel me down endlessly
unfolding cold corridors,
icy tile flecked in black
leading toward the scans
where magnetic eyes
try to find the bloom behind my
garden walls of bone,
the hidden gray flower,
all budding mystery.
Being and brain
enfolded into shy petals
opening out to the world, softly,
moving in sensory breezes,
reaching to see.

Always they search the flower
looking for the curled brown places
left by illness's smoldering heat,
the scars disordering my visual world.

For now, at times, I perceive
only fragments in a scene.
They show me a photo from a magazine—
glossy confusion—till—
there—a kettle—hence—a kitchen.
Connections between things
melt away as if objects exist alone
in isolation.
Pulled under white waves
lost among things,
i feel myself receding, sometimes.

Then in the quiet time of twilight
as i watch red-and-orange become
transmuted into pink and lavender,
two images come to me.
i weep to see the first:
my flower, wilted, in places
withered and dry.

But as my tears flow, the image
dissolves into a second.
I see my dewy gray bloom
arching up from its roots
to embrace aqua sky.
The flower
pulses, perfused by love
which nourishes my soul,
coursing in unseen strength,
forever concealed from prying
blinded scanner eyes.

As I gaze out the clear glass window
to the city beyond,
twilight crosses over into darkness,
but the room remains bathed in color,
washed of whiteness
while my gray flower
closes its petals
to sleep awhile
in the gentle evening.

There was one physician, a neurology resident on my medical team, who, even as he, too, was caught up in the general excitement over the testing and my symptoms, remembered that there was a person involved, that I was more than an interesting case. He visited me often and always kept me well-informed about everything that was happening.

One day he said, "Melissa, I want you to understand that some of this testing we're performing is experimental. It may provide us with information that we can directly use to treat you; it may not. But we know so little about how lupus affects the brain. Your case might help us to learn more about CNS lupus. Eventually, hopefully, this will benefit you and others, though we can't make any guarantees. You don't have to go through with some of this testing, but it would really mean a lot to us." He was the only one to acknowledge to me that the testing, though of possible clinical use, was also being utilized as research. Instead of assuming that this was all right with me, he asked my permission, which I greatly appreciated. He made me feel more in control, less lost.

The issue of primary interest to me was treatment. The doctors thought about sending me home on oxygen, but no one, myself included, was happy about the idea. There are no side effects from receiving low doses of oxygen, but I certainly did not want to walk around with a portable oxygen tank. I had enough trouble getting about without any encumbrance straining my abilities to maneuver. And I was a young woman who wanted, as much as possible, to maintain the lifestyle of a person my age. That did not include a portable oxygen tank, usually carried by someone much older. But I was spared the tank. The neurologists decided that the problem could be addressed by medication. They concluded that the oxygen deprivation was causing seizures that could be treated by using Depakote, an anticonvulsant, and I was kept in the hospital while the Depakote built up in my bloodstream.

Dr. Averapporti decided to discontinue the cytoxan, which was no longer providing the relief that it had in the past. Also, after the last few treatments, my white cells had not regenerated as quickly as they should have. And the potential for devastating side effects from the cytoxan increased with every dose. Dr. Averapporti and I decided to try methotrexate, a milder form of chemotherapy than cytoxan. Methotrexate is less toxic with fewer side effects, but it is much less powerful. When we had wanted to blast the lupus with our most forceful ammunition, cytoxan, not methotrexate, was our drug of choice. Now that cytoxan was no longer an option, we would try methotrexate and see how I responded.

Finally the doctors discharged me. I was too weak to live on my own, so I went to my parents' house for several months to regain my strength. I took a leave of absence from school, planning to return in January. During that fall, I did improve, though my symptoms did not disappear. Though I still battled the fog, gradually, my power to write and think came back to me. I felt able to reconnect myself to the world, and in that I found comfort and hope. And the Light. I now had knowledge of the Light that could penetrate any fog, any darkness.

I was able to return to school in January, and I was grateful to be back. As always, the university felt like home. But my physical state remained unstable. Despite the Depakote, my seizures continued to be poorly controlled. I was told that I was having "breakthrough seizures," because my disease was so generally active. The methotrexate did not seem to be working. Therefore, in the spring we decided to use pulse steroids as needed in addition to chemotherapy. The IV steroids did help, though, as always, at a price. Still, at that point, I was willing to accept the side effects in exchange for some small respite. After a steroid treatment, the mists would clear for a little while and words would be mine again. I treasured my rediscovered words, turning them over in my mind as if they were jewels possessing texture, color, shape, and light.

I did not receive the pulse steroids in the hospital. Instead, a nurse came into my apartment to administer the treatments. At first I was extremely uncomfortable with this arrangement. My home was my haven, a place where I studied, relaxed, and entertained friends and family. I felt that bringing the treatment into my home was an invasion, a violation of the boundaries I wanted to maintain between my illness and my normal routine. I worried that my neighbors would see the nurse going in and out of my apartment; I would lose my privacy. Also, I tended to be sensitive to medication. What if something went wrong? In my home, I would not have the resources of the hospital near at hand. But Dr. Averapporti and his nurse convinced me to give the home infusion a chance.

I did so, with much misgiving. The nurse, Patrick, arrived. He was a young man a little older than I. I must admit that I felt awkward about having a male nurse take care of me. I had met only one male nurse in the SPU, and he looked after the male patients. As I sat on my couch, unbuttoning my blouse so that Patrick could insert the IV needle into the catheter in my chest, I almost blushed, to my surprise. I had become accustomed to disrobing in hospitals and doctors' offices. I certainly was no exhibitionist, but after so many examinations, I was no longer as modest as I had been when I first became ill.

However, I found that it was an entirely different matter to expose my body in my own home and not in the setting of the hospital. In my apartment, if a man put his hand inside my blouse, it was not supposed to be for a medical treatment! Though I knew intellectually that being touched by Patrick was in no way romantic or sexual, I remained uneasy. I realized then the powerful and important role that the setting of a doctor's office or a hospital plays in transforming a physical examination or medical procedure from what would otherwise be an intimate encounter into an asexual act.

But gradually, Patrick set me at ease. His manner was professional, and he was obviously extremely knowledgeable and competent. He was also personable and intelligent. The four hours passed quickly in pleasant conversation. Over the months, with each treatment, we got to know each other better. Though I never looked forward to receiving the drug, I did enjoy our talks. I became accustomed to receiving the treatments at home and no longer felt threatened by them. Though I did insist that Patrick take all the equipment with him when he left. I did not want to be constantly reminded of the lupus and the medications by keeping an IV pole or a needle box in my apartment. At least between treatments, I wanted to keep my apartment as free from the evidence of disease as possible.

That summer of 1994 I was awarded another internship to study with Esther. We planned to teach our course one last time in the next spring term, my last semester in the M.L.A. program. I had some serious doubts and reservations about teaching. What if I erupted into a seizure or began to twitch from the myoclonus while I was in class? The tremoring of my hands, my voice, and even my head had become much more noticeable. Though teaching was emotionally satisfying, it was also physically draining. Then I remembered my previous teaching experiences. The names and faces of former students crowded into my mind, and I recalled the many delights of teaching—the writing conferences, the lectures, and the class discussions. I also remembered my vow not to let the seizures turn me into a prisoner, barred from others and all that I could do. I was a teacher. And if it was at all possible, I was not going to allow the lupus to take that from me.

At that time, Dr. Averapporti and I decided to stop the methotrexate, which was clearly not helping me. In June we began monthly treatments with IV IG—intravenous immunoglobulin. The IG solution consists of a mixture of antibodies that, through a process not clearly understood, is supposed to prevent the immune system from producing harmful, self-destructive antibodies. The infusion was given over two days, for about four hours each treatment. The IV IG infusion did bring me relief, though the improvements never lasted more than a few weeks. And I did not gain the benefits without paying a cost. For about four or five days after the infusion, I always felt as if I had the flu. On multiple occasions, I became ill with viral meningitis as a result of the treatment. Viral meningitis is not contagious or fatal, but it is painful.

But the side effects were worth it; the treatments were effective enough so that I could return to school in the fall. That autumn was a hectic time for me, and I needed all my strength to tackle my full schedule. Esther and I were still working on our syllabus for our course. I was taking two classes, one of them a fascinating course in the history and sociology of science department. The class, "Disease and Society," was taught by the department's chairman, Professor Friedman, a noted historian of medicine. As the course progressed, I realized the different ways in which the experiences of the lupus patient and the physician treating the disease could be placed in a historical and societal context. For my term paper I decided to write about lupus. I also wanted to expand the paper into my graduate thesis. I went to Professor Friedman to discuss my ideas and ask if he would act as my thesis advisor during the spring semester. Professor Friedman had a particular interest in chronic illness; he was conducting his own research in that area. He agreed to be my advisor, with Esther as my second reader.

During that busy fall term, I was also applying to Ph.D. programs. I sent out eight applications to universities across the country. I applied for a fellowship as well. Gathering all my records, filling out the forms, taking the GREs (Graduate Record Examinations), and writing the application essays consumed an incredible amount of time. My family was generous with their time and assistance, turning my search for a graduate school into a family endeavor. My parents proofread my essays and applications. My mother handwrote information onto the application. By that time, my handwriting consisted of little more than indecipherable scratches resembling beetle tracks. My brother helped me refresh my math skills for the GREs.

Though my parents helped me in every way possible, they had serious reservations about my going forward with my Ph.D. Most of their concerns were the same as before, when I had looked at graduate schools after receiving my B.A. Ph.D. programs generally did not allow part-time students. Did I have the physical stamina to carry a full-time load? Was I in any position to move away from Philadelphia, my family, and the medical team caring for me? I knew that these were legitimate questions. But I answered my parents, "I don't know how I am going to feel in the spring or next fall. I am not going to decide now that I am going to be sick then. Lupus is so unpredictable. I may not be able to go for my Ph.D. next year, but I'm not ready to close the door on the possibility. I want to apply and have all options open to me." They felt that my approach was reasonable and realistic. All we could do was wait and see.

There were other considerations besides illness. Academia was changing, and not for the better. At Laurel University, I had been insulated from many of these upheavals, but I was informed about what was happening. The academic world I had known as a child was disappearing. My father had been a professor during the glory days of academia, when funding was plentiful and attitudes were different. Now monies for research were drying up. Competition for grants and fellowships had become fiercer than ever before. Public indignation about the cost of higher education was growing, and one bone of contention was professors' salaries. The public asked angrily, "Why should professors receive such a large salary and teach only one or two courses?" In an effort to appease the public, state universities were eliminating positions and requiring the professors who remained to take on a much heavier teaching load. This left little time for professors to conduct research. To cut costs, both public and private colleges and universities were getting rid of jobs or at least enforcing hiring freezes. In my field, literature, there were approximately three hundred applicants for each full-time teaching position.

When I sought the advice of Philip Dawson, my undergraduate thesis advisor, he was quite blunt: "If you want to get your Ph.D. because you're interested in learning more about literature, then by all means continue. But you have to accept that you will not be able to work as a full-time professor in academia. There just aren't any jobs right now. And this isn't going to change in the near future. The odds are that after getting your degree, you would have to get a job doing something else." In fact, Philip was involved with a program sponsored by the university's business school that found jobs in the corporate world for liberal-arts graduate students.

What if I spent all that time and effort pursuing my Ph.D. only to find that I could not get a job in my field when I finished? Would it still be worth it to me to stay in school? Even if I was hired as a full-time professor, did I want the position? I had always envisioned that my life as a college or university professor would consist of a harmonious balance of writing, teaching, and doing research. But in today's academic world, that seemed unlikely, maybe impossible.

Throughout the fall I wrestled with these questions. The dream of becoming a professor had been with me since childhood. It was as much a part of me as my dark brown eyes or my need and desire to write. How could I let my dream die?

I finally decided that I would not make my choice then; I would wait for the spring and consider all my options at that time. Perhaps this was simple procrastination. But I also had a sense that when the moment came, I would know what to do. In the past, all my major decisions had worked out that way. What had begun in turmoil or confusion ended in clarity and the feeling that I had made the right choice. I hoped that with the spring would come the insights I needed.

Meanwhile, the lupus continued its onslaught. At the end of October I had an attack of hemiparesis and could barely move the left side of my body. I dragged the left side with me when I walked as if it were some heavy piece of wood attached to my body. I was frightened. Despite aggressive treatment, I was still developing new neurologic symptoms. What would come next?

I was hospitalized for this flare, but for once, my mother was not with me. She and my father had left for a cruise through the Mediterranean. I stayed in the hospital for about four days. Friends brought me things that I needed from my apartment. The day after I returned home, my mother called. She woke me up, so I was a bit hazy at the beginning of our conversation. I asked, "Are you two home already?" She told me that, no, they were still on board ship; in fact, she was calling from somewhere in the Mediterranean Sea. She wanted to know if I was all right. The night before, she had dreamt that I was ill and needed her. She was terribly upset and woke up crying. Telling herself that she was being ridiculous, she tried to go about her day, but she remained unsettled.

Finally my father said that she should call me to put her mind at ease. I did not mention my hospital stay; I did not want to ruin her vacation. I reassured her that all was well. As I hung up the phone, I felt discomfited by my mother's uncanny sixth sense. She had displayed this knack before for knowing when something was wrong with me. But I didn't know her mother's intuition could reach across several thousand miles.

At long last, all the applications were in the mail, classes were over, and the "Medicine and Literature" syllabus was in order. My schedule for next semester, the spring term of 1995, was set. I would be teaching with Esther and taking an independent study with Professor Friedman in order to complete my thesis, "Systemic Lupus Erythematosus: Patients, Their Physicians, and Support Groups." I rested as much as I could over the winter vacation, conserving my strength for my final semester in the program.

I began research for my thesis with enthusiasm. After living with and reading about the illness for almost seven years, I thought that writing the thesis would be mostly a matter of compiling and synthesizing my knowledge. But months of interviewing doctors, patients, support group leaders and members, and reading lupus narratives, medical journal articles, medical texts about lupus, as well as articles from the popular media, taught me a great deal, some of it quite surprising to me.

I felt that I gained the most insight on the subject of lupus metaphors. I did not intend for this topic to become a focal point of my research. But as time went on, I realized that lupus was overlaid with meanings and metaphors integral to the experience of lupus patients and the physicians who treated them. These conceptions about lupus were as much a part of the disease as its biological characteristics.

First, I looked at the lay literature such as lupus narratives, brochures put out by the Lupus Foundation, and articles from the popular media. I found that the words "mysterious," "enigmatic," and "bizarre" are frequently applied in defining this disease, which is often called "the great imitator," because it so often mimics other diseases. The tone and choice of words used in the descriptions of lupus create the perception of lupus as lurking and strange. For example, a brochure from the Maryland Lupus Foundation features the slogan "Lupus, The Hidden Disease That Lasts a Lifetime."

A piece I read in *Good Housekeeping* was the most thorough and generally objective in tone out of all the articles from the popular media; however, even that article begins with a dramatic headline in boldface: "THE DISEASE THAT FOOLS THE DOCTORS: It's widespread, hard to diagnose, disabling—and 90% of its victims are women. Here's what you should know about LUPUS." The word "fools" underlines lupus's "sneaky" nature, and the entire title conjures up the image of lupus as an elusive, mysterious, and powerful attacker of women. This depiction of lupus is found in other articles such as "Lupus: Master of Disguise," and "Ordeal. Richard and Jeramie Dreyfuss: Hollywood's Courageous Couple. The inspiring story of their fight against a mysterious disease."

The metaphors and meanings associated with autoimmune disorders also play an integral role in the public's conception of lupus, as lupus patients' narratives make clear. On a purely biomedical level, autoimmune diseases involve the body's defenses mistakenly attacking its own tissues. But autoimmune disorders have taken on layers of meaning beyond the physiological. These diseases have become metaphors for the psyche's attack upon the body: the ill person is seen as self-hating. Of course, this metaphor increases the societal and self-blame so often associated with chronic illness.

Lupus narratives are replete with language and imagery that show the ways in which the lupus patient thinks of the disease as a form of psychological self-attack or self-punishment. Often the narratives are written in the patient's hope that, through the process of writing, self-realization will occur, the knots of self-hatred will be untangled, and the disease will come under control. *Heartsearch: Toward Healing Lupus,* by Donna Talman, and *Lupus Novice: Toward Self-Healing,* by Laura Chester, are two such examples. In her portrayal of her illness, which began with arthritis in her hands, Chester writes,

> But it was *my* move flicked the cellular switch, self-repulsion on the structural level, collapsing the castle, setting the bones on fire, exhausted under the noiseless hum. I tightened up the reins on life itself, until my hands ached as if from a horse ride. But we know the fingers were just too eager to take, that conscience doesn't want you to cheat one bit, that life is constant in its demand for you to give, and that you cannot control The World.

Did I, on some level, also believe that I had subconsciously "flicked the cellular switch"? My intellect told me that, no, I had not caused my disease through some kind of self-hatred. But I had always harbored a lingering, persistent guilt about my disease. Perhaps that sense of guilt stemmed from my early reading of Siegel and Cousins or from some of my experiences with physicians who blamed me for my disease. But maybe, without my being aware, I had internalized some of these notions about autoimmune disease. Perhaps, somewhere in my mind I did really believe that the lupus resulted from a war between my psychological self and my physical self, a battle that made me the cause of my own disease.

Another basic element in the public's conception of lupus is the identity of lupus as a skin disease. As I mentioned before, the term "lupus" had, since the Middle Ages, been used nonspecifically to describe skin conditions in which the skin of the face appeared as if it had been eaten away by a ravenous wolf. These conditions inspired fear and horror, as the name "lupus" (Latin for "wolf") attests. In the illness narrative *In Search of the Sun,* by Henrietta Aladjem, a physician from Peter Bent Brigham Hospital explains to Aladjem that skin diseases have the power even now, as in the Middle Ages, to "bring out unreasonable fears in people," including thoughts of "contagion, of curses, of filth, of evil, of unworthiness."

Until the late nineteenth century, the often systemic nature of discoid lupus (a form of lupus that affects only the skin) was not recognized. Historically, the most basic distinguishing aspect of the disease's identity was its distinctive, disfiguring rash. Only relatively recently, in the 1920s and 1930s, did pathologists discover that lupus may occur without skin manifestations. Today lupus still carries the meanings associated with skin diseases.

The metaphors and meanings that shape the conception of lupus in the general public's consciousness greatly interested me, but what I found even more fascinating was the language, imagery, tone, and metaphors physicians invoke when describing lupus. The words "mysterious," "enigmatic," and "bizarre" appear just as frequently in discussions of lupus presented in medical texts as they do in the lay literature. In fact, the language deployed by physicians to talk about lupus is often more florid than that used by laypeople. In his preface to *Rheumatic Disease Clinics of North America* (1988), John Klippel, a rheumatologist from NIH, refers to the "deranged immunity evident in lupus." "Deranged" implies the irrationality of madness. Klippel also speaks of the researcher's endeavor to "unravel its [lupus's] secrets."

In the preface to his textbook *Systemic Lupus Erythematosus,* Dr. Robert Lahita explains in a rather dramatic manner: "SLE most likely is caused by an agent(s). The agents or agent remain unknown and may be novel, but the result is a form of biologic anarchy, which throws into disarray one of the formidable systems of the body, the immune system." The overall tone suggests mystery. There are causative "agents" that are not only "unknown" but might also be new. Like Klippel's choice of the phrase "deranged immunity," "biologic anarchy" also transmits images of disorder and chaos.

Later, in the introductory overview, Lahita continues, "In essence, the fundamental rules of biological protection are violated for unknown reasons. . . . The illness affects the fundamental fabric of life like other unknown illnesses." The word "unknown" appears a total of five times in a single paragraph. Lahita also repeats the word "fundamental," first in conjunction with "violated" and then with "fabric of life." These heavily laden terms possess connotations that seem to identify SLE as almost profane— an entity shrouded in mystery, a perversion working against the body's normal physiological nature.

Physicians do seem to conceive of lupus as violating a natural order. Dr. John Stone, a cardiologist at Emory University School of Medicine, dramatically displays this point of view in his collection of essays, *In the Country of Hearts,* when he writes, "The exact cause of lupus is uncertain, but it is known that in the course of the disease the body makes antibodies directed against and damaging to its own organs. The process amounts to a kind of immunological betrayal of its owner by the body, an absolute autoimmune revolution." He calls the disease "capricious" and labels the antibodies "turncoat."

Why, I wondered, do physicians harbor such strong feelings about lupus? I could only speculate, but it seemed to me that the concept of self-destruction at the cellular level, in other words, autoimmune disease, clashes violently with what we assume to be the most fundamental and dependable biological drive—self-preservation. The human organism is geared in amazingly and wondrously complex and intricate ways toward self-perpetuation and self-protection. But lupus defies this most basic law of human biology; for physicians this signifies disorder and chaos. I argued that these attitudes about autoimmunity combined with the emotionally charged conception of lupus as a ravaging skin disorder converged to produce the current sentiments physicians implicitly, though strongly, express about lupus.

Whatever reasons lie behind physicians' notions about the disease, my research showed me that these attitudes are deeply embedded. They create a recurring theme in biomedical texts, scientific articles, papers presented at conferences, and popular articles and essays written by physicians. In my thesis, I asked how these beliefs clinicians hold about the disease itself, as an entity distinct from the patient who suffers from it, affect the way in which the clinician views and treats his or her lupus patients. I could give no definitive answer. I assumed that these notions about lupus complicate the already complex and problematic relationship between the physician and the lupus patient by feeding into the sense of frustration, helplessness, and uncertainty the physician already feels when treating this disease.

From personal experience, I had witnessed how illness metaphors, even metaphors of the lupus as wolf, could play a beneficial role. But when I finished my thesis, I also understood that lupus comes laden with various meanings, associations, and metaphors that, unfortunately, can burden both patient and physician. Though I enjoyed my research into the history of lupus, support groups, and the doctor-patient relationship, it was the language of illness and what it revealed that truly absorbed me. Though I approached my subject as a social scientist and a historian, I realized that, even in this type of study, I still looked at my topic through my poet's eye.

While I was writing my thesis, I co-taught with Esther. Teaching was as delightful as ever. True, it was now even more complicated by disease, especially the myoclonus, seizures, and tremoring. I was also experiencing cognitive problems such as difficulties with my memory, organization of my thoughts, and word recall. At the beginning of the semester, I spoke with Esther; we agreed that she would take over the lecture if I gestured for her to do so or if I appeared too shaky to continue speaking. Once during the semester, I did not accompany Esther to class. A few minutes before we were supposed to teach, I felt a seizure coming on, and I stayed behind in Esther's office. But since there were two of us teaching the course, my absence did not mean the class could not go on. Having a co-teacher made it possible for me to teach.

That spring, I took great pleasure in my teaching and my research, but more than ever before, I was having to draw on every last resource to function. I lived on Tylenol to fight the fever and pain. My anticonvulsant dosage was higher, making me groggy but helping somewhat to decrease the number of seizures. To combat the sleepiness, I ingested huge amounts of coffee. The caffeine made the tremoring worse and certainly did not do my stomach any favors, but I needed the stimulant to stay awake. On particularly bad days, I increased my oral steroids slightly. In an effort to stem the tide of disease, Dr. Averapporti began to administer a combination of IV IG and pulse steroids each month. The steroid treatments gave me just enough relief to stay in school, though the disease remained active, especially in its neurologic and cognitive symptoms. I became extremely Cushionoid. I filled with fluid and gained a great deal of weight. When I looked into the mirror, I saw a moon face peering back at me.

Dr. Averapporti and I discussed what to do next. There were no easy answers. We talked about cyclosporin, a powerful immunosuppressant used in transplantation. Imuran, another form of chemotherapy, more powerful than methotrexate, was another possibility. Dangerous side effects were issues in using either drug.

By this point, it was obvious that I could not go on for further graduate

study, at least not for the next academic year. The lupus had made my decision. I felt betrayed by my self and my illness, alone in an unlit darkness.

Finding myself on the plains,
chased there by the wolf of my illness,
I looked behind
haunted by shades of former selves.
In longing I reached to hold them in my grasp,
but they tumbled past
with the whisper of dried leaves.
Now it seems I have been trapped here
in endless stretches of time
vast as the plains,
rolling expanses of hazy present moments.
I am driven further out onto the plains
in their all-consuming flat emptiness,
with their constant night
parched by unrelenting summer heat and winds
flaying the earth, destroying the crops.

In other days, I lived peacefully on green hills,
others by my side.
There in land and sky I found my words.
I brought them inside me,
held and nurtured them, created my poems,
then sent them into the world,
part of myself born and recreated—
sustained.

On the plains, my ears bloody as I hear
the tearing winds, the baying of the wolf.
There are moments when wind and wolf
cease their howling,
but the plains remain, still barren,
devoid of words, absent of others.
And in the silence, more intensely
do I perceive my muteness.
In the stillness, more clearly
do I hear the song of lost hopes and dreams.

Then the voice of a friend comes to me
from a land far beyond;
he sends a painting made of words,
a landscape of the plains,
understanding brushed
on a canvas of compassion.
The solitude broken,
I hear the calls of others,
and my spirit lifts and follows to lush lands
where love tills the earth.
There walks a friend from childhood,
now a bride who invites me to share her joy.
I find another friend weeping in mourning.
I give her what comfort I can;
even in the midst of pain,
a friendship grows as love is offered
to ease a sorrow.
There are others who speak to me,
people I never knew except
for the words they sent to the world.
Through their passionate speech
their lives touch mine;
my spirit becomes animated
in their embrace.

So even as my body stays prisoner
in the land of wolf and dust
my spirit does not wither,
but takes root in fertile soil,
nourished, protected
from the ravaged plains.

As I had stood in the black night, a lamp had been lit as I reached out
to others and they reached out to me. My spirit had found solace and comfort. But as the semester came to a close, and I finished my thesis and taught
my last class, I still had no answers about my future. What could I do now
that I would no longer be able to travel the path I had chosen so long ago?

17

Desert Invocation

Summer 1995–Summer 1997

THEN SOMEONE called out to me. My professor, Dr. Friedman, spoke. "Melissa, I think you should develop your thesis into a book. This is excellent work. Continue with it." My family added their voices to his. My mother said, "Melissa, you're a writer, and that's what you should be doing. You have so much to give through your writing. Your father and I believe in you." As I looked into my parents' eyes, I saw their love but also their respect. Their support of my writing full time did not come out of pity or blinded love but out of a true belief in my abilities.

The memory of reciting my first poem, my little haiku about the eagle, came back to me. I watched myself standing before the class, feeling as if I had uncorked a magic bottle and released a genie holding the gifts and delights of language. Yes, I was a teacher. I hoped that I would stand in front of a classroom again someday. But first, and above all, I was a writer. I could not teach at the moment, but I could give of myself and connect to others through my writing, as I had always done. As one path had been consumed, another had revealed itself to me. I was being offered the opportunity to devote myself completely to the craft of writing.

I set my feet upon the new path that began where the old one had disappeared. At first my steps were unsteady, uncertain. As always, I took great satisfaction and pleasure in the act of writing. But I had been a part of life at a university for the past ten years. Without active involvement in an academic community as a student, a teacher, and a colleague, I felt isolated. My vital source of everyday contact with others, especially peers with the same interests, was gone.

At the beginning, my work on the manuscript could not act as a conduit of communication with others, because for the first four or five months, I was not ready to share any part of the manuscript with anyone. I spent almost two months learning to use all the new computer equipment my parents gave me. Then I needed time to organize my materials, plan an approach to my work, make outlines, and refine those outlines—all before I composed the first sentence. During that time, I worked alone.

I believed in my project and did not regret my choice to devote myself to my writing. But whenever I went to the campus for a doctor's appointment, I would see students and professors rushing back and forth, and I would feel the pain of absence, as if a limb had been amputated.

Feeling restless, one day I decided to go on one of my rambles about the city. Occupied with my thoughts, I accidentally wandered into a rather seedy section of town.

> Houses built row upon row,
> jagged teeth crumbling in urban decay.
> I hurry on my way,
> for even though the sun
> blankets the streets and banishes shadows,
> (sunlight seems to feel no fear in lingering here)
> my mother's warnings and solemn newspeople
> cast a pall over my steps.

> Then, a voice calls out (to me?),
> "My, that's a pretty cane.
> But I guess you don't use it for that."
> I pause and see a small man,
> about my height
> yet as dark in skin as I am fair.
> I stand poised for flight in case of danger
> and think it odd to hear my cane praised,
> just a metal tube with a rubber handle,
> ugly symbol to me of what I have lost.
> A puzzle.

> But when I try to see the cane
> through his eyes
> I realize that the way the sun strikes it,

the cane sparkles
and perhaps, does become a thing of beauty
like his words and friendliness,
offerings to a stranger.
I smile and thank him.
He laughs in return saying,
"Your smile just brightened my day.
Thanks for stopping.
Don't mean you no harm, you know.
Don't mean no harm."
I walk away
filled with joy and shame.

As I made my way home, I realized that I did not need the sheltering walls of the university to stimulate my mind or make contact with people. Meaningful exchanges with others were possible even in brief encounters with strangers met on the street. As I thought back, it struck me that I had always made these kinds of connections with people, but until I was completely removed from my school routine, I did not understand their significance. The world outside the university teemed with life and people. It was time for me to take full part in that world.

I returned to my writing, more at peace than I had been when I left my apartment earlier that afternoon. Over the months I began to build a new life for myself. I joined a book club for the enjoyment of discussing books with people who also derived great pleasure from reading. I applied and became a part of the NCIS—National Coalition of Independent Scholars. In this way I became a part of a learned community even though I was no longer associated with a university. And just because I had left Laurel, that did not mean I could not participate in various university-sponsored events such as talks, lectures, colloquia, and alumni functions.

I also kept in touch with certain faculty members. I had somehow thought that when I graduated, it meant that my ties with them were automatically severed. But that was not at all true. They were warm and supportive, and they continued to be interested in what I was doing. Esther chided me for thinking that our friendship would be altered by my departure from the university. Our friendship thrives, and with her encouragement, concrete advice, and guidance, she has played an integral role in the writing of this book.

Eventually the book served as a way to establish contact with others. Friends and family members contributed to my project with enthusiasm and generosity, offering their suggestions and sharing their own memories of events. A new friendship has grown out of my work. I first met Jean in an English class we were taking while students together in the M.L.A. program. After Jean graduated, she also began writing a book, and over the months, we exchanged our work and gave each other advice. But our relationship has gone far beyond professional discussions of our writing. She has become an important person in my life, one whose friendship I treasure.

And so I find that two years have passed since my graduation in the summer of 1995. I have continued on in this new life I have created, one that is rich and fulfilling. The wolf still walks with me. He is the assault on my body. He is the onslaught on my spirit. And he is the attack of the physicians when they blame me for my disease. It is the last manifestation of the beast that I cannot yet accept or even completely comprehend, though I have gained much insight over the years. I do not know how to fight against the wolf when he comes to me in this form or how to completely let go of the anger I feel when I think of how he has ravaged me in this way. The savagery of his attack this past winter especially preys upon my mind.

It is the middle of August, and I have brought my troubled thoughts with me on a trip to the beach, where I am spending a few days with my parents. My parents have packed many of the same fears and questions, as well as their own anger, in their suitcases. It seems that the three of us have come with heavy baggage indeed.

It is early evening, and we are walking on the quiet boardwalk, away from the crowds near the amusement park. I walk slowly, hesitantly, dragging my stiff, spastic left leg behind me, trying to keep my toes from catching in the uneven boards. I lean heavily on my Canadian crutches. The ugly armbands, metal covered with gray rubber, wrap around my arms like shackles. My legs are rigidly enclosed in the unyielding plastic of my braces. Finding a bench underneath a pavilion, we stop so that I may rest.

We talk about a new radical lupus treatment that my parents have read about in the newspaper. They want me to find out more information and consult Dr. Averapporti. The treatment involves many risks, but we are ready to explore it even so. My parents and I are accustomed, from long experience, to dealing with severe flares of my disease and partial recoveries. But it is now eight months since the latest flare began, and despite aggressive treatment in terms of medications and physical therapy, I have not been able to make the kinds of gains I always have in the past.

I cannot yet exchange my crutches for the straight cane I used before this December, but physical therapy has discharged me, believing that, at least for the moment, we can make no more progress. I cannot walk more than a block or two and must rely on my scooter for longer distances. I am grateful to have the machine because it allows me to live on my own. It takes me to the grocery and the drugstore, and its roomy baskets carry my packages. In this way, I can keep myself supplied with the basic necessities of life. When the fog in my mind lifts enough for me to work, I can go to the library on my scooter to do research for my writing. I still go on my rambles throughout the city, but it is by scooter, not on foot.

Though the scooter brings me independence of a kind, it is more limited than that which I enjoyed before December. My life is regulated by the weather. I cannot ride the scooter in the rain or when the sidewalks are not completely clear of snow or ice. When the scooter needs repairs and cannot be used, I am trapped, dependent on others. Many places are not accessible by scooter. When I am home, I see my straight cane gathering dust in the corner. How I once hated that cane, unpleasant reminder of all I could no longer do. Now, roaming around the city with only my cane, no crutches or scooter, would be delightful. The cane has become a symbol of recovery.

The Dilantin levels have not been under control, because Dilantin or one of my other drugs has put my liver into overdrive. Though I have not had a grand mal seizure since February, when the Dilantin level drops or the lupus becomes more active, I have partial seizures. I do not lose awareness during these episodes, but I cannot control the left side of my body. Unlike the grand mal episodes, there is no warning, no aura before the partial seizures. So I do not have the time to get myself to a safe place before the seizure begins. Because these partial seizures take me by surprise, I often fall when they occur.

My parents have frequently witnessed this new type of seizure. About two months ago, when I was spending the weekend with them, they went out for awhile. On their return they found me sitting on the steps leading to the second floor. I was recovering from a partial seizure that overcame me as I was heading up the stairs. At that point my parents decided that I should go back to my apartment, where there are no steps. Though my being alone during these seizures petrified them, it was better than taking the risk of my tumbling down their staircase and being seriously injured or killed in the fall.

A bottle of codeine is now in my medicine cabinet, and I carry a supply
of tablets in my purse. I do not leave for a vacation without the drug. Never
in nine years of illness did I keep a narcotic in my house, employing other
methods to fight pain. But now my old ways are not always enough to
control the pain that visits me daily. All of this my parents know.

They wonder and worry now more than ever before. Will I be able to
go further in my recovery? What will we and my doctors do if I flare again?
What medical options are left? Will the drugs harm me as greatly as the
disease? How long will I be able to continue living on my own? In the event
of my parents' death, how will I cope financially? Who will provide for me
then if I cannot do so for myself?

Though my parents are relatively young, in their early fifties, and suffering from no life-threatening illness, I know that these last two questions
haunt them. They have mentioned several times how they have set up their
wills so that I will be protected financially if they are gone. This has been a
family concern. My grandparents, Bubbe Pearl and Zaide, have also told me
that their wills leave almost everything to me.

These last words are difficult to write. I do not even want to think of
losing my parents or my grandparents, whom no sum of money can replace. But I also realize, though I would rather not, that my parents' questions about my future are justified. I am currently unable to work, and we
do not know when or if that will change. Though medical insurance has
covered most of my bills for hospitals, doctors, and medications, there are
many costs of living with a chronic illness for which insurance does not
pay. These expenses have only increased because of this latest flare, height-
ening my parents' apprehensions.

Discussion of this new lupus treatment and all it represents leads to my
parents' repeating their bitter, angry refrain about the horrendous care I
received in February, particularly from the neurologists. I shared their fury
over these past months, but as my parents speak, I realize that my feelings
on the subject are much more complex than they were in the early spring.
I am startled to discover that even though I have not fully released the anger
I feel toward Dr. Fields, Dr. Gresley, and all those physicians who have
blamed me for my illness, my rage has abated. I have let much of it go, bit
by bit, in the writing of these pages.

My parents have had no such outlet. As I listen to them, anguished for
their pain, I hear their battle cry against the wolf in all of his manifestations.
They can do nothing to stop the wolf from tearing at my mind and body or

to give me back that which has been taken from me. They may as well try to grasp the moon in their hands. So they focus all their wrath on the neurologists. Unlike the wolf in his other forms, the neurologists can be held accountable for their attack. And it is not entirely blind or displaced anger which directs my parents. They are right to blame Dr. Gresley for her label of pseudoseizure, a diagnosis which became such an obstacle in my receiving the care I needed during my hospitalization in February. Dr. Fields should be held responsible for his refusal to acknowledge and treat the grand mal seizures I experienced in rehab.

Dr. Gresley's and Dr. Fields's actions might have had serious, even deadly, consequences. If the ER doctor had not intervened, the steroid toxicity would have been dismissed as stress-induced shakes, because, after all, I was a hysteric who dealt with anxiety through pseudoseizures. If Dr. Daniel, Dr. Averapporti, and Dr. Lighton (the neurologist we consulted for a second opinion) had not insisted on prescribing Dilantin to control the seizures, I might have experienced uncontrollable grand mal seizures at home. Judging from my current sensitivity to Dilantin levels, it is quite likely that would have happened. As a result of these seizures, I might have broken bones, suffered brain damage, or died.

But when my parents blame the neurologists for the steroid toxicity, I know that they are holding the physicians responsible for something that no doctor could have foreseen. My parents believe that Dr. Gresley and Dr. Fields should have realized in October that removing the anticonvulsant would increase the steroids to a dangerous level. If only the neurologists had been paying attention in the fall and decreased my steroid dosage then, I would not have become toxic on the steroids later. I would be recovered by now.

I, too, wish that I could blame the neurologists for the steroid toxicity, for the ground I have not yet regained. I would possess an explanation more satisfactory and reassuring than the idea that this past flare and toxic reaction were unpredictable, unpreventable events. I would feel more in control, less at the mercy of my medications and my disease. But sometimes, even if physicians do their job well, making no mistakes, illness rages on, medicines wreak havoc on the body, and it is not the physicians' fault. No one is to blame. Not them. Not me.

I ask my parents to be just by not holding the neurologists accountable for what was nothing more than my bad luck that I could not tolerate the steroids and that the lupus flared again. But my parents, tortured by their grief, cannot hear me. They go back to the house, but I stay underneath the pavilion on the boardwalk, watching the ebb and flow of waves on the shore as the sun settles lower in the evening sky.

As I sit, I think of how my parents' inability to cope, at this time, with what they cannot understand or control makes them lash out in a way that is not completely rational or fair. With a startled indrawn breath, I realize that my parents are behaving exactly as so many of my physicians have done. With a rush like the waves coming toward me, I understand the full meaning of the wolf, the beast in his shape as the attacks from physicians who have blamed me for this disease.

Except for the specialized skills and knowledge they have acquired, physicians are no different from my parents. Or me. Or you. As I learned long ago, they are not the angels, devils, or omniscient demigods our society often believes them to be. They are mere humans—parents, daughters, sons, brothers, sisters, friends, lovers, husbands, and wives. Like patients and their families, physicians often feel profoundly disconcerted and powerless as they face this illness which is filled with mystery and uncertainty, this disease which doctors frequently cannot comprehend or subdue.

In my master's thesis, I wrote extensively about illness metaphors and the language physicians use in describing lupus. I analyzed how their words and images reveal their deep-rooted dread of this disease. I even recognized that their attitudes toward the disease, as an entity apart from the patient, could further burden a physician in caring for a lupus patient by increasing the physician's already high level of frustration. But somehow, I never connected these concepts in any fundamental way to how I thought and felt about my own victim-blaming experiences.

My mind turns to Dr. Averapporti, who flippantly remarked during one of my last office visits, "Treating you has been so traumatic, we should both go in for therapy. Except I couldn't afford it on what CGH pays me." Through black humor, he revealed the pain he felt about all I endured because of this disease and his inability to keep the wolf, in all his guises, from me.

So many other physicians along the way have given me glimpses into their own inner struggles. I remember the neurology resident who took such great delight in the improvement of the spasticity in my hands, because he felt that he only diagnosed patients' problems and never actually did anything useful for them. And the plea of my current neurologist, Dr. Lighton, who after giving me new medicine, wanted me to call him, even if I experienced relief and no side effects. "We need to know when we have done well and helped our patients," he said seriously. His words took on added depth and poignancy when I looked into his kind brown eyes, which fully expressed how much he wanted to help me.

But physicians, like patients and their loved ones, can become trapped in their own pain, unable to deal with the emotions they feel about the illness. When this happens, they begin to blame their patients. And I believe that these doctors only feel worse after doing so, though they will not admit to themselves what they have done and why they have done it. After my hospital stay in February, Dr. Averapporti encountered Dr. Fields. Dr. Fields, looking regretful, asked Dr. Averapporti about me. My former neurologist made no excuses for himself or his department, but Dr. Averapporti felt that Dr. Fields was saddened over the way our relationship had ended and that he missed me.

Dr. Averapporti's account brings back memories of Dr. Kostos. Several years after Dr. Kostos left me to crawl around on the hospital floor, I met with his nurse coordinator to interview her for my graduate thesis. At the second interview, she said that she had mentioned me to Dr. Kostos. He wanted her to tell me that he was thrilled to hear of my continuing with my education and that he wished me well. In my anger and hurt, I had dismissed both Dr. Kostos's and Dr. Fields's responses as insincere, unimportant.

But as I sit in the pavilion, gathering all my memories, they assume their proper place and meaning. I realize now that many of these physicians who place such a burden on their patients do not come away unscathed. These doctors who cannot cope suffer not only for what they feel but also for how they behave. Like me, they bear their own inner scars.

They, too, are victims of the wolf.

I have found my own ways to keep myself intact and whole while traveling with the wolf. Physicians who treat lupus, or any chronic illness, need to do the same. Ideally, their medical training should help them develop ways to cope with treating chronic illness. Instead, their socialization into the profession only makes it more difficult. Physicians are taught not to accept either their own limitations or those of present medical knowledge, boundaries with which they frequently come into contact as they treat their chronically ill patients.

Instilled into physicians are the following basic expectations: the physician must be able to explain the cause of illness with certainty and precision and be able to cure or at the very least control it. To diagnose and cure, or at least control, illness: this is what it means to be a doctor in both the

medical world and in our society. But for doctors who treat chronic illnesses, it is like chaining them to a rock which they are told to push uphill,
yet they have no hope of reaching what has been defined as the pinnacle of
success. When they can no longer deal with the strain of pushing that rock,
physicians blame patients.

Success? Failure? What do these terms mean for the physician who
treats chronic illness? These concepts must be redefined by medical educators and by society, so that physicians stop blaming their chronically ill
patients. In treating chronic illness, the doctor cannot cure. But he or she
can improve the quality of the patient's life; the physician can and must
find fulfillment and take pride in that accomplishment. Again I think of
Dr. Averapporti. In the rheumatology office, there are three folders, each
several inches thick, holding the history of my disease and of all Dr. Averapporti's attempts to make the disease submit. In terms of cure, or even
control, those pages document his failure. But *I* do not view him or his
efforts as a failure, and I do not want him to either.

Because of Dr. Averapporti's care, I have been able to go forward with
my life in all its fullness, reaching many of the goals I set for myself. Obtain-
ing my B.A. and my M.L.A. Writing this book. He administered medicines
that, while not curing or providing any lasting control, diminished my
symptoms enough so that I could go on. While he could not prevent my
becoming disabled in various ways, he made sure that I received the help
I needed to remain independent and continue with much of what I had set
out to do. He acknowledged that chronic illness invades both body and
spirit, and, without blaming me, introduced me to Dr. Cohen, my psychiatrist, who could tend to those wounds that went beyond the physical.

Even when Dr. Averapporti could do nothing else, he always traveled
with me, bearing empathetic witness to my struggles with the wolf. I will
never forget coming to see him when my mind was shrouded in the mists.
I attempted to tell him what I was experiencing, but I could not. He remained silent a moment, then, touching my hand, he said, "Did you ever
see the movie *Charley*? It's like that, isn't it? When Charley starts to lose
his powerful mental abilities, the most terrible part of it is his awareness
of what's happening to him." I felt soothed and calmed. Dr. Averapporti,
through his understanding, had reached into the imprisoning, isolating fog
and given me the companionship and support I so desperately needed.

Dr. Averapporti makes no secret to himself or to me of his limitations,
both those of his own knowledge and those of medical science. He accepts
the many uncertainties inherent in treating chronic illnesses. He accepts his

own flawed humanity. In doing so, Dr. Averapporti defines his identity and role as a doctor in a way that allows him to cope with treating chronic illnesses, blaming neither himself nor his patients for those things beyond his control or understanding. He is no longer chained to a rock, condemned to pushing it uphill to an unreachable destination. He is free to be the kind of healer chronically ill patients need. As a physician and a healer he succeeds.

These insights bring understanding, but they do not erase the culpability of Dr. Gresley, Dr. Fields, or the others. These doctors are still accountable for what they have done. No matter what forces act upon us, I do believe in each individual's free will to act. With that freedom comes responsibility. There is no forgiveness in me for Drs. Gresley and company, for those particular individuals. Not yet. Maybe never. But, still, I know now what I must do. I must relinquish my anger, for it brings me nothing. It is only a burden I have carried, my heart's heaviness. With these last words, I lay it down, leaving it in the desert sands. As I rise from the ground, I find compassion and hope reign in the place where anger once ruled. Compassion for all the victims of the wolf, including physicians. And hope that by sharing my understanding, I may keep some physicians from striking out at their patients—and themselves.

I began with the following invocation:

> **May my pen be the confessor of sins, and you, my reader,**
> **the priest. May the doctors who are in need of it**
> **find mercy and absolution in our efforts.**

I would end with this invocation:

> *May my pen bring healing to us all—physicians,*
> *patients and their loved ones, and to you, Reader.*
> *May we all find healing from the beasts we encounter*
> *along our path.*

Epilogue

September 1997

AS I FINISH writing those last words of the manuscript, the letters on the page take on a grainy quality and become like so many bits of sand. They coalesce to form a complete picture of the desert, not a flat snapshot but a living image. I hear the desert winds and almost feel the heat of the sun. And the river. There, beside the river's shores, I see myself. And I know the river's source at last is near.

The picture begins to shift, and it is as if I watch a film contained within the borders of the page. I have the sensation of being both outside the unfolding scenes and a part of them. I feel in control of the direction I will go, and yet I also sense that I am being led.

As the Melissa inside the film stands by the river's edge, she—I—hears a faint sound, a soft yet steady pulse. Puzzled, I follow it. As I travel east, walking toward the sound, the light of the rising sun becomes ever stronger. This light does not burn. I only sense warmth and illumination emanating from it. Eventually I reach the place from which the river flows, a sacred space of green, emerald against the pale flesh of the desert. At the center grows a rose, its crimson petals velvet soft and dewy, sustained by the river, the lifeblood of this desert land.

I lean closer to inhale the flower's exquisite scent, and as I breathe in the delicate perfume, the sound and scent enter my being and the words "grace and beauty, joy and meaning, love given and love received" appear in my mind. Other words are whispered in tantalizing phrases I cannot interpret. The words are of a language beyond human understanding. I realize then that I have found the beating heart of the desert land. Enduring bloom secreted at the center. Revealer of all things, yet keeper of mysteries unknowable.

In celebration I lift my head to the rising sun whose rays caress the desert flower, the river, and me. Then once again, I set my feet on the road east, the wolf beside me.

I watch the Melissa on the page walk off into the distance, until I can see her no more. I close my manuscript and travel on.

Notes

For additional information about lupus, the Lupus Foundation of America and the Arthritis Foundation are excellent resources. If you prefer online services, I recommend the "Lupus around the World" Web site at www.mtio.com/mclfa (sponsored by the Lupus foundation) and the "Hamline University Home Page" at www.hamline.edu/lupus/.

Prologue

Illness Narratives

. "That is what those who had come before me had done . . ." p. 2

Before 1950, book-length personal accounts of illness were rare. Since that time, illness narratives (as well as memoirs in general) have proliferated. What is the character of this evolving genre, the child of the late twentieth century? What are the most common ideas, themes, motifs, structures, and images in illness narratives? As a group, who are the authors? What are their backgrounds? The two intertwined questions that follow intrigue me the most. First, why, in this latter half of the twentieth century, have such a large number of people felt compelled to communicate their experiences of illness in this way? And why has there been such an eager audience waiting to hear the stories these authors feel the need to tell?

I cannot answer these questions in this note. These queries deserve book-length responses and the scholars Anne Hunsaker Hawkins (*Reconstructing Illness: Studies in Pathography*) and Arthur W. Frank (*The Wounded Storyteller: Body, Illness, and Ethics*) have done just that. Their analyses are far from exhaustive, but they are beginnings in the academic study of the new genre of illness narratives. Another excellent resource in examining the subject of illness narratives is the Medical Humanities Database sponsored by NYU. Their "Literature and Medicine" section offers a list of illness narratives. This is by no means a complete bibliography, but it is an interesting and helpful compilation. The journal *Literature and Medicine,* published by Johns Hopkins University Press, is also a good resource for articles about illness narratives.

I will not attempt a long or detailed discussion of illness narratives. However, I feel that within the context of this genre, I must more fully explain my rejection of the "we shall, and did, overcome our disease and regain our good health" plot lines of the illness narratives to which I was mostly exposed, especially in the early days of my illness. I do not wish to be misunderstood. *I am not stating that this is the character of all illness narratives.* But in my experience, it is the most popular kind of illness narrative. And unlike other kinds of illness narratives, for me, such accounts are ultimately destructive, not empowering, as they are meant to be.

In her study of illness narratives, or pathographies, as she calls them, Hawkins identifies certain organizing themes, "central myths" in her terminology, that appear in many illness narratives. These myths include battle, journey, rebirth, and "healthy-mindedness." As I define it, the theme "we shall and did overcome" in illness narratives is equivalent to the myth of "healthy-mindedness" Hawkins describes.

"Healthy-mindedness" is a term Hawkins borrows from William James. At the turn of the century, James described what he saw as a growing movement sweeping over the country. The "religion of healthy-mindedness," according to James, was associated with a general relentless optimism, as well as the more specific views that nature is inherently and absolutely good, evil and sin are illusions, and positive emotions conquer all. For those blessed with healthy-mindedness, the world is ruled by a beneficent Nature in which living right means loving others, being happy, and using one's mind to think optimistically. In contrast, the "sick soul" (defined by that soul's feelings of fear, guilt, despair, and belief in the intrusion of evil in the world) cannot maintain a healthy-minded attitude; it is impossible for it to do so, a flagrant distortion of its reality (127).

Hawkins argues that the religious attitudes James wrote about one hundred years ago are strikingly similar to the medical versions of healthy-mindedness—especially the same wellspring of uplifting optimism. Hawkins cites three basic, defining aspects of healthy-mindedness in health care today. First, psychological and emotional factors are emphasized in the cause and treatment of illness. Second, there is a powerful belief in the body's ability to heal itself. Last, active involvement of patients in all aspects of their treatment is emphasized. Sick people are responsible for becoming ill, usually by their lifestyle, stress, feelings of unresolved anger and depression, and they are also responsible for getting well again (128–129). Norman Cousins's *Anatomy of an Illness* definitely comes to mind.

As I discovered mainly by experience, so Hawkins found through her research. For she writes that "attitudes and behaviors associated with healthy-mindedness are evident in many pathographies published in recent years." Later, she even uses the term "entrenched" to describe the popularity of this particular myth in illness narratives. She goes on to say that the myth has become so entrenched that "it already has its detractors in the pathographical literature" (148), though their numbers are still relatively small. I am not the only one to feel burdened by what Hawkins terms the myth of healthy-mindedness, which I call the persistent drumbeat theme "we shall, and did, overcome" of so many illness narratives.

Chapter 6

Victim Blaming

"As I later learned from my own experiences as well as those of other lupus
patients, it is not at all uncommon for a physician to blame the victim when
the diagnosis is unclear."   p. 84

In *Travels with the Wolf,* I show the havoc that victim blaming can wreak, and I call
for healing and reform. But my views on the subject have grown from more than just
my own encounters with health-care professionals. I have been a member of the lupus
community for the past ten years and have come to know many other chronically ill
patients. While I was an undergraduate, I started a lupus support group at my university. Also, through referrals from my rheumatologist's office at CGH and from the local
AJAO (American Juvenile Arthritis Organization) chapter whose meetings I attended,
I counseled young adults and sometimes teens who were chronically ill with lupus or a
different rheumatic disease. Over the past ten years, I have also participated as a member
of the Philadelphia and Delaware Valley chapters of the Lupus Foundation of America,
attending support group meetings, symposia, and lectures. Then there are the countless
others I came to know in many different ways—chronically ill persons with whom I
shared the wait in a doctor's office or perhaps the confines of a hospital room. I often
listened to these people's stories of their own experiences with physicians. These chronically ill individuals' spoken narratives shaped the opinions I present in this book.

My perspective also derives from my research as a graduate student. In my master's thesis, "Systemic Lupus Erythematosus: Patients, Their Physicians, and Support
Groups," I used the tools of sociology (especially interviews and participant observations) and the history and sociology of medicine to study victim blaming (thesis 3, 13,
17, 47). In the context of the doctor-patient relationship the phenomenon is complex;
it is rooted in the history of medicine and in our culture. Sociology and the history and
sociology of medicine gave me formalized, objective tools with which to study victim
blaming. In writing *Travels with the Wolf,* I tried to bring together the "objective" information and analysis I had gained through my graduate research with my own "subjective" experiences and impressions. Hopefully, the parts have formed a greater whole.

Chapter 7

The History of Lupus

"The name 'lupus' in association with the disease now known as systemic
lupus erythematosus evolved over centuries, beginning with Hippocrates."
p. 95

I found Sheldon P. Blau and Dodi Schultz, *Lupus: The Body against Itself* (Garden
City, N.Y.: Doubleday, 1984), 20; Nathan J. Zvaifler, ed., *Rheumatic Disease Clinics of*

North America (Philadelphia: W. B. Saunders Company, 1988), 4; Robert G. Lahita, ed., *Systemic Lupus Erythematosus* (New York: John Wiley, 1987), 2; and Daniel J. Wallace and Bevra H. Hahn, eds., *Dubois' Lupus Erythematosus,* 4th ed. (Philadelphia: Lea and Febiger, 1993), 317, very helpful in describing the history of lupus.

Lupus as Wolf

> "But I think the most vivid and creative lupus-as-wolf imagery can be found
> in cyberspace . . ." p. 94

The use of the lupus-as-wolf image on the Internet is worthy of a much longer discussion than that given in the text or in a short note. I was overwhelmed by the amount of data when I went surfing on the Web. But there were a few additional examples that I wished to mention. "The Wolf's Den" is the name of AOL's (America on Line's) support group. Two other Internet support groups, "Lupus HOPE1" and "Lupus HOPE2," contributed to the online collection "Poems and Personal Reflections Written by Our Members," which is filled with references to the wolf. Sometimes the wolf is sneaky or senselessly cruel, as in the lines, "I was bitten by a wolf / I don't know why." Another sufferer entitles her poem "My Friend the Wolf."

In "The Lupus Book Forum," a Geocities Web site, the wolf runs rampant in this compilation of stories, poems, and other creative works by people with lupus. A few of the titles: "My Dance with the Wolf," "Sleeping with the Wolf," "Wolf," "Wolf in the Shadows," "My Wolfbit," "Some Days You Get the Wolf, Some Days the Wolf Gets You!"

There are two Web pages in particular whose intricacy and complexity fascinate me. "Kathryn Ann's Wolf Writer's Home Page" and "Forestgreen's Wolfden" are both completely organized around the theme of the wolf. In both, the names of the locations in the Web site reflect the wolf motif: "Wolf Angel" and "Wolf Recovery Foundation Site" in Kathryn Ann's page and "Learning to Walk with the Wolf" (an account of her experiences with rehab) in "Forestgreen's Wolfden." On Forestgreen's page the decoration along the top and sides of the screen consists of actual photographs of various kinds of wolves. Also, to go from location to location, one must click on an icon of a wolf baring its fangs. Kathryn Ann's relationship to her wolf is unusual. Though she abhors her wolf and grieves over its coming, in another sense, she sees the wolf as a spirit guide, a kind of totem—a view for which she reaches back to her roots as a Native American.

Chapter 13

Poem Citation

> Some say the soul can be found
> pulsing in the heart.
>
> p. 190

This poem, "Hands," originally appeared in *JAMA: The Journal of the American Medical Association* 269 (March 10, 1993): 1240.

Chapter 16

Lupus as Metaphor

> "But as time went on, I realized that lupus was overlaid with meanings and metaphors integral to the experience of lupus patients and the physicians who treated them."   p. 244

In the quote above, I am referring to the experience of writing my master's thesis in 1995. I explain how I come to my conclusions by looking at the lay literature such as lupus narratives, brochures put out by the Lupus Foundation, and articles from the popular media as well as the professional literature written by and for physicians (medical texts and journal articles, etc.). There are a few points I would like to address.

First I must make an update. The most recent (1996–1998) materials written about lupus and distributed by the Lupus Foundation of America, the local Philadelphia chapters, and the national organization, have changed. Though the idea of lupus as an unpredictable mimic of other diseases is still present, it is no longer a major theme. Brochures, fact sheets, and texts like Mary Moore, ed., *Learning about Lupus: A User Friendly Guide,* 2d ed. (Delaware Valley chapter), are optimistic in their outlook, emphasizing that lupus can usually be controlled, though not cured, through proper treatment. What is known about the disease is highlighted, rather than what is unknown. The matter-of-fact and often upbeat language of the brochures reflects this change in attitude. The material is stripped bare of such words as "mysterious," "enigmatic," and "bizarre"; lupus is no longer termed "the great imitator." The difference between the tone and language of this literature from the LFA and the literature I reviewed for my thesis is marked.

I am fascinated by this change. Obviously, I cannot explain the reasons behind this, or even fully document it in this note. Research, particularly interviews with LFA health educators, would have to be done to uncover the answers. To make an obvious point, the new brochures are much more reassuring to the patient and his or her loved ones, particularly when the ill person has just received the diagnosis of lupus. Perhaps this was the goal of the LFA.

Susan Sontag might argue that the absence of metaphors in the LFA literature signifies an increase in knowledge about lupus, for she asserts that the less known about an illness, the more people create metaphors to fill the void. But that is too simplistic an answer. Though some strides have been made in increasing our understanding of lupus, the basic questions about the disease remain unanswered. What is its cause? How can it be absolutely diagnosed? How should it be treated? What is its prognosis? How can it be cured? We still do not know.

Also, the metaphors live on in other areas. Informally, I have continued to keep track of metaphors in lupus narratives, articles from the popular media, and materials written by physicians. As far as I have been able to tell, these still contain the metaphors I found in 1995. Lupus has become better known over the past few years; it has appeared with increasing frequency as the subject for the lay and professional writers. I would have much more material to work with than I did for my master's thesis. I would be intrigued to delve into the subject again, to see how the central metaphors and meanings of lupus have changed, if at all, since 1995.

Two key works informed my writing about illness metaphors. Susan Sontag's *Illness as Metaphor and AIDS and Its Metaphors,* was one, of course. The other was Emily Martin's *Flexible Bodies: Tracking Immunity in American Culture: From the Days of Polio to the Age of AIDS.* In her work, Martin explores the pervasiveness and power of immune-system imagery and its associated ideology, both in the scientific world and in the general public. She does not probe deeply into the meanings of autoimmunity. But she provides strong evidence to show that scientists and lay people alike view the breakdown of this part of the body with special horror and dread.

Bibliography

Below I list those materials to which I refer in the text and in my notes as well as a few additional important works on the subjects of chronic illness, the training of health professionals, lupus, and illness metaphors. I did not include the full bibliography from my graduate thesis. Even if I had done so, this bibliography would not be, and is not meant to be, a literature review, for those as well as other topics discussed in *Travels with the Wolf*.

Aladjem, Henrietta, and Peter Schur. *In Search of the Sun*. New York: Macmillan, 1988.

Aronowitz, Robert A. *Making Sense of Illness: Science, Society, and Disease*. Cambridge: Cambridge University Press, 1998.

Arthritis Answers. Atlanta: Arthritis Foundation, 1998.

Bell, Linda. *The Red Butterfly: Lupus Patients Can Survive*. Brookline Village, Mass.: Branden Press, 1983.

Blau, Sheldon P., and Dodi Schultz. *Lupus: The Body against Itself*. Garden City, N.Y.: Doubleday, 1984.

Breedlove, Charlene, associate editor, *JAMA*. Interview by author, November 1992.

Bridgeman, Erica. "Waking Up with a Wolf in My Bed." *LIFT Magazine* [online] 1.05 (June–July 1996).

Camus, Albert. *The Plague*. 1948. New York: Vintage Books, 1972.

Charmaz, Kathy. *Good Days Bad Days: The Self in Chronic Illness and Time*. New Brunswick: Rutgers University Press, 1991.

Chester, Laura. *Lupus Novice: Toward Self-Healing*. Barrytown, N.Y.: Station Hill Press, 1987.

Cousins, Norman. *Anatomy of an Illness As Perceived by the Patient: Reflections on Healing and Regeneration*. 1979. New York: Bantam Books, 1985.

"The Disease That Fools the Doctors." *Good Housekeeping*, April 1992, 60+.

Fibromyalgia Syndrome. Atlanta: Arthritis Foundation, 1997.

Fox, Renée C. "The Human Condition of Health Professionals." Lecture delivered at the University of New Hampshire, Durham, N.H., November 19, 1979.

———. *The Sociology of Medicine: A Participant Observer's View*. Englewood Cliffs, N.J.: Prentice-Hall, 1989.

Frank, Arthur W. *The Wounded Storyteller: Body, Illness, and Ethics.* Chicago: University of Chicago Press, 1995.

Goldstein, Melissa. "Medicine and Poetry: A Pathway of Communication." *The Pharos* 61 (1997): 12.

———. "Systemic Lupus Erythematosus: Patients, Their Physicians and Support Groups." Master's thesis, University of Pennsylvania, 1995.

———. "William Carlos Williams: The Physician as Writer." Bachelor's thesis, University of Pennsylvania, 1992.

Hawkins, Anne Hunsaker. *Reconstructing Illness: Studies in Pathography.* West Lafayette, Ind.: Purdue University Press, 1993.

I May Look Okay . . . But I'm Not. I Have Lupus. Baltimore: Maryland Lupus Foundation.

"Illness Narrative/Pathography." A list of illness narratives available from the literature and medicine Web site at New York University.

Katz, Robert S. *Steroids in the Treatment of Lupus.* Rockville, Md.: Lupus Foundation of America, 1994.

Klass, Perri. *Other Women's Children.* New York: Random House, 1990.

Kleinman, Arthur. *The Illness Narratives: Suffering, Healing and the Human Condition.* New York: Basic Books, 1988.

Klippel, John. Preface to *Rheumatic Disease Clinics of North America,* ed. Nathan J. Zvaifler. Vol. 15, no. 1. Philadelphia: W. B. Saunders Company, 1988.

Kübler-Ross, Elisabeth. *On Death and Dying.* New York: Macmillan, 1969.

Lahita, Robert G. *What Is Lupus?* Rockville, Md.: Lupus Foundation of America, 1998.

———, ed. *Systemic Lupus Erythematosus.* New York: John Wiley, 1987.

Lassett, Barbara. *Lupus, Stress and What Doctors Don't Tell Us.* Great Neck, N.Y.: Todd and Honeywell, 1986.

Lewis, Kathleen S. *Successful Living with Chronic Illness.* Wayne, N.J.: Avery, 1985.

Lundberg, George D., M.D., editor-in-chief, *JAMA.* Interview by author, November 1992.

Lupus: A Guide to Diagnosis and Treatment. Atlanta: Arthritis Foundation, 1997.

"The Lupus Book Forum." Web site. Link at www.geocities.com.

"Lupus: Master of Disguise." *Current Health,* December 1989, 26–27.

Mann, Thomas. *The Magic Mountain.* 1924. New York: Random House, 1969.

Martin, Emily. *Flexible Bodies: Tracking Immunity in American Culture from the Days of Polio to the Age of AIDS.* Boston: Beacon Press, 1994.

Moore, Mary E., ed. *Learning about Lupus: A User Friendly Guide.* 2d ed. Ardmore, Pa.: Lupus Foundation of Delaware Valley, 1997.

"Ordeal. Richard and Jeramie Dreyfuss: Hollywood's Courageous Couple." *Ladies' Home Journal,* November 1988, 100, 109–10.

Permut, Joanna Baumer. *Embracing the Wolf: A Lupus Victim and Her Family Learn to Live with Chronic Disease.* Atlanta: Cherokee, 1989.

"Personal Home Pages on Lupus." [online]. Links available at the Missouri Chapter of the Lupus Foundation of America (MCLFA). Web site at www.mtio.com/mclfa/.

"Poems and Personal Reflections Written by Our Members." [online]. From the support groups Lupus HOPE1 and Lupus HOPE2. Available at members. aol.com/pentweelie/poems.htm.

Percy, Walker. *The Moviegoer.* 1988. New York: Ballantine Books, 1990.

Raveche, Elizabeth S., and Alfred D. Steinberg. "Systemic Lupus Erythematosus." *Encyclopaedia Britannica: Medical Health Annual,* 1988. 505–8.

Rosenberg, Charles E. *Explaining Epidemics and Other Studies in the History of Medicine.* New York: Cambridge University Press, 1992.

———, and Janet Golden, eds. *Framing Disease: Studies in Cultural History.* New Brunswick: Rutgers University Press, 1992.

Rosenthal, Elisabeth. "The Wolf at the Door." *Discover,* February 1989, 34+.

Sacks, Oliver. *The Man Who Mistook His Wife for a Hat and Other Clinical Tales.* 1970. New York: Harper and Row, 1987.

Selzer, Richard. *Confessions of a Knife.* 1979. New York: William Morrow, 1987.

———. *Down from Troy: A Doctor Comes of Age.* New York: William Morrow, 1992.

———. *Imagine a Woman and Other Tales.* New York: Random House, 1990.

———. *Letters to a Young Doctor.* 1982. New York: Simon and Schuster, 1983.

———. *Mortal Lessons: Notes on the Art of Surgery.* 1974. New York: Simon and Schuster, 1987.

Shem, Samuel. *The House of God.* 1978. New York: Dell, 1988.

Siegel, Bernie S. *Love, Medicine and Miracles: Lessons Learned about Self-Healing from a Surgeon's Experience with Exceptional Patients.* 1986. New York: Harper and Row, 1990.

Solzhenitsyn, Alexander. *Cancer Ward.* 1968. Harmondsworth, Sussex: Penguin, 1971.

Sontag, Susan. *Illness as Metaphor and AIDS and Its Metaphors.* New York: Doubleday, 1978.

Southgate, M. Therese, M.D. "The Cover." *JAMA* 276 (July 10, 1996): 84.

Stone, John. *In the Country of Hearts: Journeys in the Art of Medicine.* New York: Delacorte, 1990.

———, senior contributing editor, *JAMA.* Interview by author, November 1992.

Talman, Donna H. *Heartsearch: Toward Healing Lupus.* Berkeley, Calif.: North Atlantic Books, 1991.

Wallace, Daniel J. *The Lupus Book: A Guide for Patients and Their Families.* New York: Oxford University Press, 1996.

———, and Bevra H. Hahn, eds. *Dubois' Lupus Erythematosus.* 4th ed. Philadelphia: Lea and Febiger, 1993.

William Carlos Williams: The Doctor Stories. Edited by Robert Coles. New York: New Directions, 1984.

Wordsworth, William. Preface to *Lyrical Ballads*. In *Prose of the Romantic Period*, ed. Carl Woodring, 49–72. Boston: Houghton Mifflin, 1961.

Young, Roxanne K., associate editor, *JAMA*. Interview by author, November 1992.

Zvaifler, Nathan J., ed. *Rheumatic Disease Clinics of North America*. Vol. 14, no. 1. Philadelphia: W. B. Saunders Company, 1988.